# PRAISE FOR
# REGRESSION

"Any reader interested in autism experiences, diagnosis, and life changes must include *Regression* on their reading list . . . it's guaranteed to dispute popular perceptions and snap assessments of autism's reality."

—D. Donovan, Senior Reviewer, Midwest Book Review

"Her ability to set a scene and sustain a natural and oftentimes humorous voice in the face of difficult times keeps the reader rooting for her . . . She manages to make an informative text both easy to read and entertaining."

—Independent Book Review

*Regression*

by Twilah Hiari

© Copyright 2018 Twilah Hiari

ISBN 978-1-63393-742-0

All rights reserved. No part of this publication may be reproduced, stored in a retrieval system, or transmitted in any form or by any means—electronic, mechanical, photocopy, recording, or any other—except for brief quotations in printed reviews, without the prior written permission of the author.

Published by

◤ köehlerbooks™

210 60th Street
Virginia Beach, VA 23451
800-435-4811
www.koehlerbooks.com

# REGRESSION

## TWILAH HIARI

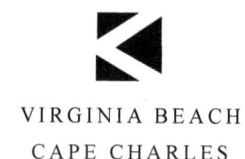

VIRGINIA BEACH
CAPE CHARLES

# CHAPTER ONE

*Jesus loves the little children. All the children of the world. Red and yellow, black and white, they are precious in his sight. Jesus loves the little children of the world.*

I LOVED SONG time. I pushed out my chest to make my voice big so that Jesus could hear me over the voices of the other kids.

Song time was over now, but the verse kept playing in my head. The plastic chair under my butt was hard, and the light shining in stripes through the blinds was bright. Miss Teacher was saying something about how Jesus commands us to love everyone like they're our brothers and sisters. I'd been told I had a brother. My mother said the screaming creature in the bayonet was a brother. I only had the vaguest idea of what *brother* meant. The piercing cries that came from the bayonet made me run outside to hide.

I listened to Miss Teacher say how Jesus said I was supposed to love everyone like I loved the creature in the bayonet, but I didn't love that creature at all. It was loud. Its skin smelled like puke, poop, and cigarettes. Everything in the house smelled like cigarettes, but when you put puke and poop smells on top of cigarette smells, it's too much. I didn't want to go anywhere near the creature.

"Twilah," said Miss Teacher, "pay attention." I looked up from my desk. I'd been holding my gaze on my Big Chief Tablet while contemplating the mysterious bayonet creature and its even more mysterious relationship to the lesson. The other kids were lined up at the classroom door. I stood and placed myself at the end of the line.

Miss Teacher opened the door, and the class filed down the hallway. Along the walls of the church preschool hung coloring book pages of Baby Jesus and Wise Men and David and Goliath and Samson. Samson was knocking down pillars.

I broke into a run to catch up with the kids in front of me. They were much bigger than me, and they were always leaving me behind. "Come on, shrimp!" yelled David. David was always yelling at me.

I tried to go faster, but one foot caught on top of the other. I crashed to the floor. "Derr! Derr!" David yelled as he slapped his limp-wristed hand against his shoulder in the universal kid symbol for retarded. "Go hang out with Ryan, you 'tard!"

Miss Teacher rounded the corner, and the rest of the kids followed. Then they all disappeared from sight. I lay on the floor and cried for a moment before pushing myself up and returning to the classroom. I needed to finish thinking about Jesus and the brother creature. I wanted the carton of chocolate milk and the animal crackers I knew the other kids were eating, but I had to solve the problem in my mind first. Back in the classroom, Ryan the Retard sat with his special teacher. Ryan got a special teacher because if he didn't have someone to watch him, he'd bang his head on his desk. Miss Teacher had told us that he did that because he was autistic. I banged my head sometimes too, but I knew to do it at home, in private, not in our preschool class, where everyone could see me.

"Aren't you going to snack time, Twilah?" Ryan's teacher asked. She was giving him slices of apple. The apple looked good. My stomach growled.

"No, I'm not hungry," I answered. I stared at my Big Chief Tablet and thought hard about Jesus and the brother and the bayonet.

Thoughts churned and churned, but I couldn't get them to unlock the mystery.

Miss Teacher was back now, and the rest of the class trailed behind her. David kicked a leg of my chair as he walked past. I kept my eyes fixed on my tablet.

Miss Teacher wove among the tables, laying fresh coloring sheets in the center of each one. I leaned forward and reached for a page. The girl to my right did the same, and her hand touched mine as I clasped a sheet between my fingers. I yanked my hand back like I'd been burned. I waited until the other three kids at the table had their pages, then I carefully removed the top sheet from the pile.

The red plastic box in the center of the table held crayons. I needed a dark yellow one to color the lions who were prancing up the ramp to Noah's Ark. As I sifted through the box, little bits of wax worked themselves underneath my fingernails. All the yellow crayons were broken. I needed yellow for the lions. I couldn't use a broken crayon. The bits of wax were pressing, pressing, pressing under my nails. The lions on the ramp to the ark stood cold and white. I couldn't help them with a broken crayon. Tears started to fall onto the page. Drops landed and oozed outward. One drop covered a giraffe's head, another wet the bottom of Noah's dress.

"What's wrong, Twilah?" Miss Teacher's hand was on my shoulder. I shrugged myself out from under her grasp.

"The yellows are broken."

"They still color the same," she said as she handed me a stub of crayon.

I regarded it. It wasn't the right yellow for a lion. It was too light. And she was wrong. Broken crayons *did not* color the same. The tearstain expanded from the giraffe's head into the boundary of a nearby cloud. The page was ruined. A small cry rose up in my throat.

"Shh," said Miss Teacher as she handed me a new page and a pristine blue crayon. "Here's Jonah and the Whale."

I took the crayon from her and examined it. It would work for the whale. "What do you say?" she prompted.

"Thank you," I answered.

I sat and worked the wax out from under my nails before I began to color.

Miss Teacher returned to the front of the class. My ears picked up bits and pieces of the lesson. "Satan is bad. Satan wants our souls."

"I love Satan!" The words flew from my mouth.

"What?" Miss Teacher's voice was shrill.

"I love Satan!" I repeated.

The rubbery feet of the chair of the girl to my right made an elephant trumpet sound as they skidded across the floor away from me.

"Twilah! You don't say that!" Miss Teacher's mouth hung open, and the other kids started making indistinct sounds. *Squeaky-talky sounds*, I thought.

I stared at the whale that I'd striped with blue lines. Miss Teacher had said earlier that Jesus wanted us to love everybody, but now she was angry because I was saying I loved Satan. There had to be a mistake somewhere. "I love Satan!" I tried again.

"You have just earned five minutes in time-out! We do not say we love Satan!" Her voice sounded wobbly, and her face was bright red.

"Why not?" I asked.

"Because Satan is bad. Very bad. We hate Satan."

Her face was as red as Ryan's apple. She looked like the cartoon pictures of Satan I'd seen, only without the pitchfork! My giggles transformed into gigantic laughs. My whole body was laughing. My feet stomped on the floor, and my hands slapped the table.

I hope that answered your question, doc. That's the first memory I have of my mind working differently from the minds of other people.

**Explain to me what happened.**

You don't see? It's so obvious. The teacher had just told us that morning that Jesus commanded us to love everyone, and then she was up there saying Satan is bad. So, I had to test the first premise, because Jesus' advice had struck me as really bad. I had to be clear on whether we really had to love everyone, because loving everyone didn't make any sense. I didn't love my loud baby brother, and I didn't love bullies like David. The teacher had given me the perfect opportunity to test what she'd said, so I did. And I didn't get why she was upset with *me* about it. I wasn't the one up there saying shit that didn't make sense. Furthermore, she couldn't explain why I had to love everyone, and everyone, which I thought meant every freaking one, somehow didn't include the devil. Then she's gonna act like *I'm* a bad kid when *she* can't explain how to make sense of that mess.

*Does that make sense in the context of your other assessments? Is that what you all would consider an autistic thought process?*

Yes, it does, and it certainly is.

I climbed the big tree in the front yard and straddled my favorite branch. I stared out across the neighborhood, taking in the yards, fences, and passing cars. I watched as Candy the neighbor lady came home from work and let Daisy the Doberman into the backyard. My mom and Candy used to be friends, but they'd stopped talking when my dog Snuffleupagus had jumped the fence and gotten Daisy knocked up. I knew now that *knocked up* meant having puppies.

After counting two blue cars, three blue trucks, two red cars, one white car, one white truck, five green cars, and one green truck, I'd tired of my view from the tree. I climbed down to the lowest branch and dangled, my hand gripping the bark as my feet hovered a couple of feet off the ground. When my hands started to feel sore, I dropped down.

Back inside the house, I watched my mom lean over the bayonet. "I'm getting ready to feed your brother, then I'm gonna fix some hot dogs for dinner."

"Okay," I said. "Why's he get to sleep in the bayonet?"

"It's a bassinet, not a bayonet," she corrected me.

Whatever it was, I wanted one. I wanted to be enclosed when I slept. My dream was to have a sleep pod like the people on *Battlestar*

*Galactica*. Maybe I couldn't have that because I didn't live in a spaceship yet, but surely I could have a bassinet. We had one in the house right now.

After a dinner of hot dogs and canned corn, I went to my room. I rolled up tight in my blankets until I knew that anyone looking wouldn't be able to find me. It was in my sleep pod for the time being.

Burt must've come home that night, because when I woke up, he was at the dining room table, eating a plate of eggs. "Morning, hon," he said in his soft voice.

"I had a dream about a giant last night. He was really super big. He wanted to eat me, but I cut off a piece of my thumb and gave it to him and he was happy. He didn't want to eat all of me after that. My thumb was enough."

"That's disgusting." Mom's voice came from the kitchen, where she was scrubbing the egg pan. "Don't talk about stuff like that."

I climbed onto a chair. I swung my legs beneath me and bounced a bit, excited that my dad was home. "I wrote a story about a rabbit."

"Did ya, hon?" He stood and took his plate to the kitchen, where he placed it in the sink. From there he headed to the living room, where he sat down in his big chair. The TV blared, but I focused on my dad. I grabbed at his leg, and he lifted me onto his lap.

"The rabbit was eating a carrot, and he saw an airplane, and there was a letter from Benjamin Franklin on the airplane about how rabbits could make lightbulbs run from the energy of the waterfall, and the rabbit went to his butterfly friends to help him get on the airplane . . ." Burt craned his head around me to see the television. The man on the TV was saying something about Iran and hostages. I jumped from his lap, threw myself on the floor and pounded it with my fists. "I hate Iran!" I screamed.

What I really hated was how the TV was the center of my family's universe. It was an ugly wooden box that spewed loud, meaningless sounds. Everything important that happened in our house happened in front of the TV. My mother reveled in telling the grand story of the TV. "That TV was hit by lightning, and it still works!" she'd cheer. The tale had sealed the television's divinity.

But Iran stuck in my mind as the object of my hatred, and for the next few weeks, every time I got angry, I thought about Iran, and every time I heard about Iran, I got angry.

Every morning, my mother helped me pull on my elastic-waist pants and snap the pinchy pearl buttons on my plaid cowboy shirt. I was now six years old, and I still couldn't dress myself. The dressing ritual took place in the living room as the heads on the TV babbled from the far wall. Mom double tied the bows of the laces in my tennis shoes, because if they came untied, I'd sit and scream after trying and failing to retie them. Then she'd hand me my metal lunchbox, and I'd walk the two blocks to school.

One afternoon, after the final bell rang, I stood against the brick façade of the school building. I glanced up from the sidewalk and saw two dark-brown-skinned girls walking in my direction. I recognized the hair of one of the girls from my first-grade class. The second girl's hair looked like the first's, but the girl was taller. *Must be her sister*, I thought.

The first girl, Latricia, marched up and planted herself inches away from me. The blue plastic barrette at the tip of her fat braid swung toward my face. I pressed myself against the wall behind me. "Are you an Oreo?" she asked.

"What?" I asked.

"Are you an *Oreo*?" she shouted.

I inched to the side, trying to get out of the range of the bits of spittle that landed on my nose as the words exploded from her lips.

"Are you mixed?" yelled her sister.

I stared at Latricia's braids as I played the strange words back in my mind.

"You're just ashamed to be black!" declared the big sister. She spat on the ground near my feet before turning and walking away. Latricia trailed behind her.

I pushed my body even harder against the bricks of the school and tried to catch my breath. I stared at the circular drive until I saw Mom's green, wood-paneled Oldsmobile station wagon pull up.

"Mom, Latricia and her sister asked if I was an Oreo. Then they asked if I'm mixed. What's that mean?" I asked as I climbed into the car.

"Latricia? What kind of name . . . sounds like stupid black girls. Just ignore 'em. This is what happens when they bus 'em in," my mother snapped.

Mom and her few white lady friends complained a lot about kids being bussed in. I wondered what was wrong with the buses. I usually walked to school. Mom only picked me up if we had to go somewhere after school let out. But I thought the field trips we took on the big yellow buses were a lot of fun. *I must be wrong*, I thought. *Riding the bus must be a very bad thing.*

I stood in front of the long mirror at the end of the hallway and examined my face. My lips were puffy—like a black girl's. I pulled a lock of hair between my fingers and stretched it straight. I pulled it down past my nose. If only it would stay straight like the hair of the pretty girls. I opened my fingers, and the lock sprung back to a coil. My hair was defective. No one else in my family had hair like mine. I turned sideways and looked at my body. Thin. Mom called me *Skinny Minnie*. But my butt was puffy like my lips. I felt my nails biting into the palms of my hands. Why did my butt have to be so puffy? Why did my lips have to be so puffy? The pretty girls had thin lips, and they didn't have bubbly butts. My butt had come from my mom, I knew. Dad was always calling her bubble butt.

It was all too much. I shrieked and ran to my closet. I burrowed in the back and pulled the clothes on the hangers toward me until I was covered. I stuffed more clothes into the crack at the base of the door to stop the light from seeping in. I howled and howled, blowing my nose into the clothes that sat discarded in my hamper. I hated my rough, curly hair that trapped the comb. Hated my big butt. Hated the pretty blonde girls at school who bounced their hands off of my head and ran away screaming "Afro" and laughing. The closet door flew open. "What are you bawling about now? I can hear you all the way in the living room, and I'm trying to watch my show!"

My mother stared down at me.

"I hate my hair. I hate my hair. I hate my hair. I hate it. Hate it!" I cried and slammed my fists against the wall.

"Well, that's the hair God gave ya, so stop yer crying. And stop hitting that wall!"

"I hate it!" I stared at my mother's hair. It was bone straight and yellow gray. I'd watched her comb it and had tried to imitate her. The comb had hurt when it'd gotten stuck in my coils.

The answer popped into my mind.

"Am I adopted?" I asked.

"No! What kind of question is that? You came out of my body. I can show you your birth certificate, little missy! Now stop your bawling, and get out of that closet. I've never seen such a crybaby in my life. It's the waterworks over every little thing with you. Go outside and play!" She grabbed me by my arm and pulled, and I stumbled to my feet.

"But why do I look different?" I persisted.

"Because your grandfather was a full-blooded Cherokee Indian, and your grandmother was Black Irish. You got the recessive genes—it's science! You look just like your grandfather. He was dark—a real Injun. I've told you this a hundred times. I'm gonna hide a tape recorder in this house and record you. Then I'm gonna play the tape back and make you listen. Then you'll understand what I go through every day with you. You'll know how stupid you sound! How you repeat things. The same things over and over! Like a broken record. Driving me crazy!"

I threw back my head and screamed. I wanted to meet my grandfather who looked like me—my grandfather with the recessive genes. I wanted to see a face that looked like mine. I wanted to know I belonged in this family.

"I can't deal with this!" my mother screamed back. "I gave up a voice scholarship to marry Burt and have you kids, and this is the thanks I get. What are you bawling about now?"

"I want my grandpa!" I wailed.

"That's why you're screaming? He's dead, honey. He died before you were born." Her voice was softer now. She folded me into her arms and sniffled into my curls.

*Beyond being mixed—just socially—how did you get along with other kids when you were in elementary school?*

Wait, you've gotta understand that being mixed *always* mattered—there was no separating that socially. But I'll try to answer your question. I wasn't good at any of the playground games. The games were segregated too. The white girls only did three things: Jumped rope, played hopscotch, or clustered in packs and talked. I got tangled up in the ropes whenever I tried to jump. I couldn't understand the hopscotch rules or hop inside the lines, and whenever I tried to join a cluster and talk, the white girls would just walk away from me. The black girls played jump rope and handclap games. I didn't even try to jump rope with them. They did fancy stuff like double Dutch and that was way more complicated than the regular jump rope the white girls did, and I'd already failed at the white girl version. The black girls would stand near the building and chant and clap their hands. I liked how the chants sounded, and I wanted to learn them, but Mom always talked bad about the black kids who were bussed in. She talked bad about their moms too. She said their moms always had bunches of kids with bunches of different dads. I believed what my mom said about black girls being bad. So, I didn't try very hard to be friends with them.

There were boy games too—kickball, dodgeball, and basketball. I tried kickball maybe twice, but the boys stopped letting me on the field after I kept swinging my foot and missing the ball or kicking the ball in the wrong direction. I didn't know which direction I was supposed to kick it. The boys somehow magically knew, but nobody had ever explained it to me. Dodgeball sucked because it was agonizing when the hard, red ball hit me in the face, so I didn't play that. And basketball, as fun as that looked, was only for black boys. The basketball boys had Afros like mine. They plucked them with gigantic picks that they stored in their hair or in their back pockets.

As enticing as the boys' games looked, I couldn't join them either. I spent my time circling the playground, inspecting ants, spiders, and butterflies. Or I'd pace the playground while making up stories in my head about the galaxies I was gonna explore one day. Sometimes I just sat and ate dirt. I liked dirt. At home I snacked on the soil from Mom's potted plants. Dirt was good.

Mom pulled me onto her lap one night as the theme song from *M\*A\*S\*H* played in the background. She opened a book and explained that it was time for me to learn how babies are made. I stared at the illustration of the pink colored man and woman, but I couldn't hear very well over the sounds of the helicopters that came from the sacred broadcasting box.

"The man puts his peanut into the woman's pajamas," Mom said.

I envisioned Mr. Peanut from the jar that my dad was always eating from and giggled. I knew it would tickle if Mr. Peanut got into my pajamas. I pictured him dancing up and down my stomach, tapping his cane near my belly button. Tears formed in my eyes, and my laughs turned to wheezes. I was dying now. Mr. Peanut was killing me.

Mom put out her cigarette in the bright-blue handmade ceramic ashtray my older brother had sent from the boys' home where he lived. She squeezed a blast from my inhaler into my mouth. The metallic taste stuck to my tongue, and my wheezes transformed into breaths again.

*Did your mother or father talk to any professionals about your unusual behavior and developmental delays?*

I don't think of Burt as my father anymore. I think of him as my fake dad. He was an over-the-road truck driver, so he was hardly ever home. I do remember one time, when I was in third grade, they took me to see a shrink. The shrink sat across from us at a gigantic desk. I don't remember the conversation, but I know he gave me pills. The pills tasted horrible, and I hid them under my mattress instead of taking them. But they didn't take me to see anyone else after that. But, do you think it mattered? Who the hell was diagnosing little mixed girls with autism in 1980?

*I looked over your grades from elementary school. They're very inconsistent. Why is that?*

When I was in class with a bully who beat me up, I skipped school. If I got a class without a violent bully, I went to school. I mean, I always got bullied, but it was worse when I had a bully who used their hands instead of just their words. When there was somebody who was beating me up on a regular basis, I'd just tell Mom I had a stomachache and she'd let me stay home. She always seemed to believe me, and I wasn't really lying because my stomach did hurt most of the time. But my grades? Whenever I had a teacher who let me do my own thing, I got good grades. But whenever I had a teacher who made me do what the rest of the class was doing, I failed. And I just didn't understand math. Math was always my nemesis.

"Mrs. Williams said to give this to you," I handed Mom the sealed envelope my second-grade teacher had given me.

"Are you in trouble? You're gonna end up just like Glen. Don't think you can't end up in state custody like him, in a home. They've got girls' homes too," she threatened.

I stared at the thick double knots in the laces of my tennis shoes. Mom talked about Glen all the time. He was supposed to be a brother, but I didn't know him. The bayonet brother, Jeffrey, was bigger now. He waddled around the house smashing plastic cars and trucks together with his hands. I wondered if my brother Glen was sleeping in a pod or smashing trucks in the boys' home Mom was always talking about.

Mom stuck her finger into the envelope and ripped it open. Her eyes scanned the paper she pulled from inside it. "They want to put you in talented and gifted! And they want you to skip third grade." She paused. "I'm so proud of you, baby girl!"

She reached down, and I stiffened as her arms wrapped around me.

The principal's office was a tiny room attached to the secretary's office.

"Now, I think starting Twilah in TAG is a good idea," Mom declared. "Her older brother was in TAG. Both of my older ones are smart. They were both reading the newspaper by the time they were four years old. But I don't think she should skip third grade. She's not mature enough. She's always crying about something, bawling her eyes out. Did you see that *60 Minutes* episode about the kids who skip grades?" She paused for a breath. The principal made a sound like she was going to speak, but Mom kept going.

"Most of those kids ended up being delinquents. I saw it! And I know my psychology! Her older brother's a delinquent—pulled a knife on me when he was four years old, and he superglued Twilah's T-shirt to her back when she was a toddler. And Twilah's small for her age. That's because of her immune deficiency. It stunted her growth. She didn't even start getting teeth until she was two! All of my kids are oddballs. It's like *The Bad News Bears*!"

Mrs. Williams and the principal looked at each another. "Well, Mrs. Muller, if you don't think Twilah's mature enough to skip third grade, then we'll just advance her like normal. She'll start TAG next Wednesday," the principal said. I stared at the ruffles on the front of her shirt. They looked like seashells. I liked seashells.

In the car, my mother shook a long brown More cigarette out of the pack and lit it. I watched the two long streams of smoke shoot from her nostrils. The smoke made me think of dragons, and the dragons made me think of wizards, and wizards made me think of King Arthur and the magic sword Excalibur.

"They think I don't know my psychology. I know my psychology." Mom's declaration interrupted my fantasy of drawing a glowing golden sword from a scabbard at my waist and slicing the guts out of the kids who tormented me at school.

My feet were cold and wet, and the bones in my fingers hurt. I heard what sounded like dogs barking my name in the distance. *Twi-*

*ruff! Twi-ruff!* I opened my eyes. My fingers were wrapped around the chain links of a fence. The neighbor's Chow Chow was barking in my face. I spun and ran back across the street to my house. The transition from the wet grass to the bumpy asphalt shocked me out of what remained of my slumber. Mom's head poked out from the screen door. She was shouting my name.

"There you are! Get in here. You're staying in my bed for the rest of the night. I can't have you sleepwalking all over the neighborhood." She walked outside in her robe and pulled me into the house.

Whenever Mom caught me leaving the house in my sleep, she forced me to sleep in her bed for about a week. Mom left the lamp on her bedside table on. I stared at the wall past the foot of the bed. It was covered in pandas—pandas from magazines, pandas on black velvet, pandas from calendars, cartoon pandas in cartoon bamboo forests. Unopened packages containing small plastic toy pandas lined the top of the dresser. I began to count and fell asleep around the time my eyes landed on the forty-second panda.

While I liked counting the pandas, I didn't like lying in the hard bed that smelled like menthol and nicotine. Mom would always lift up her shirt and make me coat her back in gooey Icy Hot cream before she turned over and went to sleep. The smell stuck in my nose. I'd wash my hands over and over in the small bathroom that was attached to Mom and Burt's room. When I'd gotten as much of the Icy Hot off as I could, I'd sit down on the toilet and pull one of Burt's *Hustler* magazines from the rack on the floor.

I would stare at the pictures of naked women. They were all thin with big boobs. Some had patches of hair between their thighs. Others had hairless folds. I read the letters and articles in the magazines too. They were about how men grabbed women with big boobs. Sometimes the women who got grabbed were secretaries. Sometimes they were waitresses. Sometimes they were lawyers in tight skirts and jackets. Every time the men grabbed the women, they would come. The word appeared over and over. *Come.* In my mind, I pronounced it like *comb*. It clearly didn't mean the same thing as when I told my dog to come, so it had to have a different pronunciation. The men liked to come a lot. I wasn't sure if the women did too, because in the stories the women were always screaming.

I decided I should stop wearing my cowboy shirts with the snaps and start dressing like the women in the magazine. That's what boys liked. If I dressed how boys liked, maybe they'd stop punching me and start coming with me instead.

The next day, I tied the bottom of a T-shirt in a knot so that it rose just above my belly button. I dug into my dresser and found a pair of pants from the previous year when I'd been in second grade. I'd learned to dress myself in the summer after first grade. I squeezed into the pants and inspected myself in the hallway mirror. I was satisfied that I looked like a magazine girl. I slid on my sandals and walked to school.

My teacher, Mrs. McMillan, pulled me aside as the rest of the class was going to recess. "What are you wearing?" she asked.

"Clothes," I answered.

"No. Why is your shirt tied up like that?"

I felt my face get hot. I didn't know how to explain about the magazine girls. "I don't know," I said.

"Well, untie it right now."

"Okay." I fumbled with the knot but couldn't get it undone. She reached down and untied it. "Now go on out to recess."

I ran out the door and down the hall toward the playground.

"The principal called me today," Mom said as I sat down at the kitchen table with the bag of Cheetos I'd scavenged from the snack drawer in the kitchen. "She said you went to school dressed like a slut. I knew you'd turn out like this. Watch. You're gonna end up pregnant by the time you're sixteen." She stared at me for a moment before turning and walking away. I heard the door to her bedroom close, and I knew she'd gone to bed. When she got upset, she'd go to bed and stay there for hours. Sometimes she'd stay there for days.

Burt came home that weekend. I heard their voices murmuring behind the closed door of their bedroom. I pressed my ear against the door but couldn't make out any words. I gave up and went back to my room. I turned my attention to my favorite book, *A Wrinkle in Time*. I looked up when the door to my room swung open.

"Your mother said you need a spankin' for goin' to school like you did." Burt was standing in the doorway holding a brown leather belt.

I was confused. I thought I was supposed to go to school. Whenever I told Mom I had to stay home because of my stomachaches, she always made me go back after a couple of days. Now, Burt was going to spank me for going to school!

I pondered the conundrum the whole time I was over his knee. The belt stung my butt and the backs of my legs. My face became wet from my tears and the snot that leaked from my nose.

"Aw shush. I ain't even hittin' you that hard," Burt said. "Crybaby."

His scolding made me cry even harder. I snorted the snot back up into my nose and started choking. Burt stood me up, and Mom came running over with my inhaler.

"I hate you!" I screamed. "I hate both of you!"

"You were an accident!" Mom yelled. "I could have aborted you, but I didn't. And this is the thanks I get!"

I pulled up my pants and ran to my room. I shoved my way through the pile of stuffed animals, books, and clothes until I reached a back corner of the closet. I held my knees to my chest and cried as I rocked gently. I'd show them. I searched around the floor until I found a belt. It was a canvas belt for wearing, not a leather belt for spanking—just what I needed.

I looped it over the rod that held the clothes on the hangers. I stood on my tiptoes and tried to fit my head inside the loop. I couldn't quite reach high enough to bring my chin into the circle. I pulled a chair from my desk to the closet. I stood on it and tried again. I knew from a movie I'd watched with my mom that you had to put your head in the noose and then kick the chair away to die. But the belt kept coming loose from the rod. I couldn't get it to tighten around my neck. I sank back to the floor and cried myself to sleep.

Not until years later did I figure out why I'd been spanked. It took me that long to understand that it had happened because of what I'd worn to school.

# CHAPTER TWO

*I ALMOST DON'T know what to say to that. Your early childhood was, I'll say—disturbing. Let's move on. How did you do in middle and high school?*

Aw, jeez. Middle school was the same old, same old—intermittent ass beatings from my classmates and a handful of friendships that never lasted. I struggled academically, because the classrooms only had partial partitions instead of walls and doors, and the noises from each class flowed into the next. It was really hard to hear.

And when I was thirteen, the shit hit the fan, as my mother would say.

Mom had been yelling at Burt off and on for the past ten years, but 1989 is the year she dropped her big accusation.

Our electricity started getting turned off, and Burt would get mad when he came home and couldn't turn on the lights.

"It's not my fault. I don't have enough money to pay all the bills and take care of your kids too. You take all that road money to wine and dine that tramp you have out in Vegas!" Mom yelled one day.

This would become a constant refrain.

"I leave enough money to pay the light bill, Debbie. I don't know what you do with all the money I give you," he answered before slouching off to his pickup truck and driving away.

Each time this happened, Mom would pack me and Jeffrey into the station wagon and drive downtown. We'd stand in a long line at the electric company, and Mom would argue with the woman at the window and then hand over a check to get the lights turned back on.

I don't remember Mom and Burt announcing that they were getting divorced. I just realized one day that Burt hadn't been home for a few months, and that was a long time, even for an over-the-road truck driver. People, animals, and things often disappeared from the house, and I never knew why. My older brother, Glen, had disappeared, my dog Snuffleupagus had disappeared, and the two small dogs that lived in the kennel in the backyard had disappeared. Now Burt had disappeared. It usually took me awhile to notice, but when I did notice, there were no signs left of whoever or whatever had formerly been there.

I knew that if my mother's pattern of behavior surrounding disappearances held out, after a year or two of silence, she'd begin complaining to anyone who'd listen that Burt had done something horrible prior to his disappearance.

I missed Burt's CB radio more than I missed him. The radio had sat in the smallest room of the house, a room they called the den. I'd go in the den on the nights I couldn't sleep and turn the radio on. I'd turn the channel knob until the voices of truckers filled the room. Then I'd pick up the mic, press the button, and speak.

"Breaker, breaker one-nine. This is Leo Lion tellin' ya watch out for smokeys in the Ursa Major." I released the button.

"Is that so, Leo Lion?" said the gruff voice, tempered by a chuckle. "Where's your mom and dad, Leo? It's bedtime, hon."

"I just come around the corner into your part of the galaxy. There's smokey bears in the Ursa Major," I repeated. The truckers had always sounded grateful when Burt used the radio to warn them about smokeys.

The trucker's laugh came loud across the radio. I'd loved my nighttime talks with the truckers until the CB radio disappeared.

I scored high on some test and was invited to go to Sumner Academy. Sumner's a magnet school for kids with good academic potential. And it's a five-year high school, so I started there in eighth grade.

My first day at Sumner was hard. I'd never ridden a bus to school before. I was a little worried now that I was one of the kids being bussed in. I knew that my new classmates would be able to tell I was bad because I rode the bus. When the bus stopped at the school, I froze. The driver had to coax me out of my seat. After standing for a moment, staring up at the school, I climbed the concrete steps, passed through a heavy door, and entered a gigantic atrium. I saw a line of kids to my right and paused. "Eighth graders over here!" a voice shouted. I saw the outline of a person waving toward the line, and I took my place at the end of it.

When I reached the front of the line, a woman at a table asked me my name.

"Twilah Muller," I said. My eyes were aimed at the table.

She handed me a piece of paper with my schedule. "Go on to your first hour now." She pointed down a hallway. I looked at the paper and started down the hall. Room 112. But I couldn't see any room numbers. I walked up and down and watched as other kids strode confidently into rooms and took their seats. I noticed they were all looking up as they walked. I looked up. I could barely make out the shape of a small plaque above each door. I squinted but couldn't read the tiny numbers. I slumped against a locker and started to cry.

A man stopped and crouched in front of me. I froze. "Hello. I'm Mr. Lopez. I teach Spanish." I stared at his bright pink tie. "Where are you supposed to be?"

I held out my paper to him.

"French class! That's right behind you, my dear."

He gestured at a door a few feet away. I turned my face back to the floor and scurried in the direction he'd pointed.

Between not being able to see and not being able to hear in the large classrooms with towering ceilings, I was off to a bad start at Sumner.

There were changes at home too. Men had started showing up at the house. Every morning I got up and went to the kitchen for Cookie Crisp, there was a man I'd never seen before drinking coffee at the dining room table. I'd pour my cereal and milk into a bowl and rush back to my room. I'd stay there until it was time to meet the bus. When my digital clock read seven fifteen, I'd grab my backpack and race out the front door. I didn't want to look at the man at the table. I didn't want him to try to speak to me like the men sometimes did while I was pouring my cereal.

One Saturday morning, Mom poked her head into my bedroom. "Your dad'll be here in an hour. The school called and said you need glasses. He's gonna take you to the eye doctor."

I went to the bathroom and started to fill the tub. I always took baths. The one time I'd tried to take a shower, I'd slipped and whacked my shin against the tub. Baths felt good anyway. They always calmed me. The water that rushed out of the faucet was ice cold. Mom must not have paid the gas bill again. I splashed a little of the frigid water on myself but couldn't get so much as a whole foot into the tub. The water felt like it was burning my skin, like it was freezing my bones.

"I hate you, you fuckin' bitch!" I screamed. I ran to my bedroom and grabbed a dirty bowl from my desk. I threw it against the wall. Then I grabbed a glass and did the same thing. Shards bounced everywhere and hit my arms, face, and legs.

"What the hell are you doing?" Mom screamed.

"You fuckin' bitch!" I threw a plate at her face.

She ducked and ran down the hall. "I *will* call the police on you! Don't think I won't. They'll take you away like they did Glen."

I threw myself on the bed and punched the pillow. I didn't want the police to take me away. I knew from my mom that prisoners only got bread and water. If prisoners only got bread and water, they probably didn't get baths with hot water either.

"Are you done with your drama now?" Mom was back. "Your dad is here."

I pulled on some clothes, pushed past her, and ran to the driveway. Burt's green Ford pickup was idling near the street. I opened the passenger door and climbed in.

"Hi, hon," Burt drawled. "How you been?"

"Okay," I murmured as I wiped tears with the bottom of my T-shirt.

Those were the only words we spoke on the way to the appointment.

I sat in the big chair and rested my chin on a cold metal bar. I'd never had an eye exam before. It was hard to keep up with the doctor's instructions on whether option one or two was clearer. It was too much.

"Oh, don't cry," the doctor coached. "If you cry, you won't be able to see any of the letters.

"Okay," I said as I tried to sniff my tears back.

"Alrighty. All done," he said a few minutes later. He held out a piece of paper. "This is your prescription. The girls up front can get you all set up."

I walked back to the waiting room and squinted around until I identified the only adult sitting alone. I tentatively headed in his direction, and as I got closer I was relieved to find that it was in fact Burt.

"Here, Dad." I handed him the paper the doctor had given me. He put down the magazine he'd been reading and took the paper from my hand. I followed him to the front desk. A lady walked from behind it and started showing us the different eyeglasses. As Burt inspected the price tags, his face got redder and redder.

When we got home, he surprised me by parking in the driveway and going inside. I sucked in a breath and wondered if Mom had brought in another man while we were gone. I wondered what Burt would do if he met one of Mom's men.

But there were no men in the house. There was Jeffrey, plopped on the living room floor playing with his Hot Wheels. His straight blond bangs flopped against his forehead. Mom lay on the couch holding a cigarette in one hand and a heating pad against her stomach in the other.

"These goddamned glasses are gonna cost me an arm and a leg, Debbie," Burt proclaimed. "Whadya do with all the child support I sent ya?"

"I paid the bills, Burt. That's what I did. I'm a poor single mother now. You're out there in Olathe living high on the hog with that hussy. I'm trying to support our kids on my own."

"Patricia's no hussy. And stop yer whinin'. I send you plenty of money. I pay for the mortgage on this house an' my own house too. You go an' pick them glasses up in two weeks. I did my part," Burt said before turning and walking out.

Two weeks later I could see, but I still couldn't hear. The teachers' voices echoed up to the ceilings and back down again. By the time they reached my ears, they were fragments, small soft vowels floating amid the occasional sharp consonant. I sat at the back of each class and doodled in my notebook. I did well in the classes where I didn't need to hear. In gym class, I earned a B by substituting written reports on sports I'd researched in the library in lieu of actually participating in sports. I got a B in typing too, because the entire class consisted of duplicating the letters on the sheets in front of us. My sole A was in art exploration. In that class, I could sit alone and bring forth the brilliant colors and images that were always swirling around in my head.

Christmas came and went. I'd asked for a skateboard, but this year there was nothing. No tree, no time with Mom, stringing popcorn, and listening to Christmas carols. Nothing. Another disappearance. Food started to disappear too. The refrigerator and snack drawer now held only crumbs. Mom had gotten a job at McDonald's. On good nights, she'd bring home a bag of Quarter Pounders and soggy fries. On bad nights, we wouldn't eat anything at all.

Slowly, the mystery men at the dining room table disappeared too. Only one man remained. His name was Terry, and he lectured Jeffrey and me all the time about how easy life was for us compared to the life he'd had in the pen he'd just gotten out of.

"We're going to the truck show in an hour, Twilah. I want you to be ready," Terry said.

"I don't wanna go," I said. I'd been to monster truck shows before, and I hated them. They were loud, and the smell of exhaust and oil stuck to the inside of my nose. The last time I'd gone to one, a bearded man holding a cup of beer had yelled at me and Mom while Burt had been at the concession stand getting Pepsis and hot dogs.

"We got half-breeds here now?" he'd shouted.

I'd stared up at him. His black T-shirt was decorated with the same X that sat on top of the car from the *Dukes of Hazzard*.

Mom had grabbed my hand and pulled me away, but something about the way the man had said the word *half-breed* had made my muscles tense. I didn't understand what he'd meant, but I knew he'd been talking about some kind of badness inside me.

"I didn't ask you if you wanted to go. I told you we're going," Terry said. "Now get your ass ready, and let's go."

"No."

"Debbie, do you just let your kids talk back like this? Where I come from, this child would be gittin' 'er little ass beat." Terry's voice was so loud I felt its vibration against my skin.

"Burt did the spanking, and it never helped with her." Mom shrugged.

"Fine. Let's go," Terry said. Terry, Mom, and Jeffrey piled into Terry's truck. It was black with white patches like the spots on a dog, and it sat on huge tires that lifted it high off the ground. I watched them go, then went to my room to read. I wanted to call my one friend—my only friend, Heather—but the phone was disconnected. Mom had told me that the collect calls from Terry in prison had been expensive and that it might be awhile before she could get the phone turned back on.

Hours passed, and my stomach churned and growled. I'd read all my books several times, so I plucked a paperback from one of Mom's bookshelves. I was a quarter of the way through *The Tommyknockers* when I heard the truck pull into the driveway.

I rushed to the dining room. Mom opened the door, and Terry entered behind her. Jeffrey brought up the rear. He was swinging a toy truck in his hand and making sounds like a revving engine.

"Did you guys bring anything to eat? I'm hungry," I said.

"We ate at the show. You could've come with us, but your highness is too good to do what the family does. You don't want to do what the family does, so I guess you don't want to eat either!" Terry yelled.

"Fuck you!" I screamed back.

"Who the fuck do you think you're talking to?" he roared.

"A piece of shit," I answered. He pulled back his fist.

"Whoa, whoa." Mom stepped forward.

"Fuck all of you. I'm leaving." I headed back to my room. Terry was on my heels. I sat on my bed and picked up a shoe.

"Oh, no you don't. If you're leaving, then you'll go just as you are. No shoes. Go ahead, you spoiled little brat. Leave." He yanked the shoe from my hand.

I stormed past him. The January snow burned my feet, but I didn't care. I wasn't going back. I ran past Eisenhower Middle School and waded through the half-frozen creek behind it. I tore through woods and ran through backyards. I rang the bell at Heather's house. Her mom opened the door.

"Twilah! My goodness. What are you doing out here with no shoes on?"

"My, my, my mom's boyfriend—" I couldn't finish. Tears had already frozen to my face, and now new ones poured out, melting the rivulets of ice that had formed on my cheeks. Heather's parents let me stay at their house for a few days, but then her mom told me I'd have to go back home. I borrowed a pair of Heather's shoes and made my way back.

"Well look! Miss Priss has finally decided to come home," said Mom as I walked in the door. I walked past her to my room. She followed.

"Drop your little attitude and get in the car," she said.

"Why?"

"Just do what you're told for once," she scolded.

I was tired and confused, so I did what she asked of me. I pushed down my eyebrows when I saw we'd pulled into the parking lot of Providence-St. Margaret Hospital.

"Come on," she said as she opened her door.

What happened next is a blur. Security guards wrapped their hands around my arms as an elevator took us to the tenth floor. Then we were in an office with a man in a white coat, and my mother was telling the story she loved to tell.

"My oldest one, Glen, is a juvenile delinquent. She's on that path now. Won't do what she's told. Refuses to do things with the family. Doesn't have any friends. Sits in her room all day and reads. Screams and cries and throws things or rocks back and forth and won't speak. Curses at her own mother when she does speak. I tell ya, if I didn't have bad luck, I wouldn't have any luck at all. I love my kids, but I don't have to like 'em, and this one's turning out to be just like her older brother. I tell her, *They got girls homes too!* They just moved her brother Glen to that home out near Salina. I tell her, *They put kids like you away if they don't get their acts together!* She's always wanted attention. She was born with an immune deficiency, and she got lots of attention as a baby. Now it's out of control. She's ruining this family." She crossed her arms across her chest.

"You bitch!" I screamed. I leapt from my chair and tried to rip my fingernails across her face. The doctor held out his arm to stop me and shouted for security. The two guards were back, grabbing my arms. They half carried me to a room and pushed me toward a bed. I heard the door click locked as they left. I sat on the bed, crying and rocking until I fell asleep.

The next morning, a nurse brought me a stack of papers and a pencil. "Fill these out. I'll come back to get them before breakfast," she said.

I read the sheets she'd handed me. *Do you enjoy sports as much as you used to? Do you enjoy time with your friends as much as you used to? Do you enjoy art as much as you used to?* The list went on and on. I ripped the pages to pieces and threw them on the floor.

What did that even mean? I'd never had anything to enjoy. I'd asked for art supplies and science kits for years, but Mom had always said the same thing: "Burt doesn't want to spend money on you kids." The only activity they'd ever agreed to pay for was Girl Scouts, and that had been years ago. I hadn't even wanted to be in Girl Scouts. It had just been an excuse for my mom to be a troop leader and read the dirty parts of Judy Blume books out loud to a room full of girls. I had nothing but my books; and I'd read each one so many times, I could almost recite them from memory. I couldn't even talk to my one friend on the phone because we no longer had a phone. We had no electricity. We had no food. What the hell did those sheets mean—asking if I enjoyed things less than I had before?

I howled and punched the wall until I tired, then I went to sleep. I sat in my hospital room, rocking and crying for six days straight. Food was brought to me on a plastic tray. Each day, the doctor would come and tell me to follow him to his office. I refused to answer his questions. I didn't speak to anyone. These people were my mother's co-conspirators. They were complicit in having me jailed for her offenses.

On the seventh day, I asked the nurse who delivered my tray if I could use the phone. She said I could and led me to a phone on the wall in the hallway. I dialed Burt. "Dad? Mom got me locked up at Providence. Can you come pick me up?"

The security guards escorted me to the lobby. Burt stood near the entrance, wearing a baseball cap and cowboy boots. "Why were you here, hon?"

"Because Mom hates me. Can I come live with you?" I asked as I climbed into his truck.

"No," he answered. "Me and Patricia aren't set up for that."

When I climbed down from the truck at my mom's house, I didn't even say goodbye.

"I got a letter from the school, Twilah. You're about to get kicked out of Sumner. We have to meet with the vice principal tonight."

"Okay."

"Burt will meet us there," Mom continued. "I'm not the kind of mother who cuts a father out of his children's lives just because we're divorced. I do what's best for my kids, even if I don't like you kids sometimes. Like I've always told you and Jeffrey, I love you, but I don't have to like you." She pulled a jean jacket on over her sleeveless Guns N' Roses T-shirt. She wore jean shorts that didn't cover all of her behind. You could see all of what Burt called her thunder thighs.

The vice principal was an Asian man who wore a white shirt and black tie. After shaking hands with Burt and my mother, he spoke. "Twilah's performance in school isn't in line with what we'd expected based on her exam scores. In terms of standardized testing and IQ testing, she's brilliant, but she's not applying herself in the classroom. I called this meeting to explain that and to find out if there might be anything going on at home that could be interfering with her performance here."

Mom's chest puffed out. "Nope, we're not goin' down that road. They tried to blame me for her brother Glen's delinquency too, and it wasn't my fault. These kids are just delinquents, like in *The Bad Seed*. She's failing because she's never applied herself. She lives in her books, and then she doesn't do what she's told to do. Her head's always in the clouds. Got no street smarts. Wanders around like she doesn't know her ass from a hole in the ground. That isn't my fault. You don't get to pick the kids God gives ya."

"With all due respect, Mrs. Muller, there are some things over which parents have control. A few weeks into the school year, we sent you a letter explaining that Twilah is nearsighted, and getting glasses has allowed her to bring up her grades in typing and art. I didn't mean to offend you. Let's talk about the things that are inside our control." Mr. Shing held his hands cupped in his lap as he spoke.

Mom let out a puff but didn't say anything else.

"Mr. Muller," Mr. Shing said as he aimed his eyes at Burt, "do you have any insights into why Twilah is so disengaged from her studies?"

"I don't know. We split up last year, her mom and me. I'm an over-the-road truck driver, so I left the child raisin' to Debbie." He nodded in Mom's direction.

"What about you, Twilah? What insights do you have?" Mr. Shing's voice was gentle.

"I can't hear in class," I said.

Mr. Shing reached for a small stack of papers and started sifting through them. "Your hearing tests were normal," he said after scanning a sheet.

"This is the other thing I deal with," Mom said, "her hypochondria. It used to be that her stomach hurt all the time. She'd give herself diarrhea thinking she had stomach problems. Then she'd give herself rashes thinking she was having allergy attacks. Pooped her pants all the way up through fifth grade. Now it's she can't hear. I took her to the health department last month because she'd been whining that she hadn't been able to poop for a week. They drew blood and said there's nothing wrong with her. She'll do anything for attention. I know my psychology. These kids think bad attention is better than no attention.

"Don't you see?" She shook her finger at Mr. Shing. "She thinks faking deaf is gonna get her attention. The doctors at Providence said she's sizzle frantic, that she's got sizzlefrania. She's mentally ill, just like her brother. Her brother Glen's been in state custody since he was four years old. That's when he turned on me like a bad dog. Twilah was born sick, and she musta gotten used to all the attention she got as a baby. But she's better now, so she needs to get over it."

"Is there anything else holding you back, Twilah?" Mr. Shing asked.

I took a breath. "I just don't want anything anymore," I explained. "I wanted to be an astronomer when I grow up, so I wanted a telescope. I wanted a chemistry set and art supplies, but I never get anything. This Christmas, I wanted a skateboard, but Christmas disappeared. So, I thought about it. I thought that if I stopped wanting things, then I'd stop being sad when I didn't get them. I don't want anything anymore. I don't want to do anything anymore. That's all." I was crying when I finished, and Mr. Shing handed me a Kleenex.

"What you just said about not wanting, that's part of my religion, Buddhism. That's a lot of wisdom from a young person. But rejecting attachment doesn't mean not trying in school. Wanting to cultivate knowledge isn't the same as wanting a skateboard."

"I don't know anything about your Buddha," Mom piped, "but I do know I'm not made out of money, and these kids today are nothing but *want, want, want*. And Burt never wants to spend money on his kids."

"Now you hold it right there, Debbie. I give you money," Burt started.

Mr. Shing interrupted them. "Twilah, will you wait in the hallway while I finish up with your parents?"

A month later, Burt picked me up from Mom's and took me to a store in neighboring Johnson County to buy a skateboard. I picked out a Rob Roskopp Monster deck with a wicked blue cartoon face. I bounced up and down, slapping my hands against my hips. Then I hugged the board to my chest and smiled so hard my face hurt. After we left the store, I asked Burt if he'd take me to the library. I checked out every book they had on Buddhism. Between the skateboard and the books, it was the happiest day I'd had in years. Buddhism would continue to inspire me for almost three decades. Later in my life, I'd loosely refer to myself as Buddhist, but I would never be Buddhist in the strict sense.

I tried my best at Sumner. I'd found that running around the school track gave me the same sense of serenity as the meditation practices I'd started experimenting with. I signed up for the cross-country team.

"Don't wear your expensive shoes to the park where we run," Coach warned us. "Last year, some kids got held up at gunpoint for their Air Jordans."

I didn't have to worry about that. I only had one pair of shoes—Converse with holes rubbed in the sides from popping ollies on my skateboard. I wrapped duct tape around them to secure the remains of the canvas to the rubber soles. When the soles had worn so thin that holes had appeared in the bottom, I quit the cross-country team.

In class, I listened as hard as I could but still couldn't hear. Mr. Shing called another meeting, and this time Burt wasn't there.

"Twilah's GPA is 1.57. Sumner is for students who are committed to excellence in academics. She's going to have to go back to her home school. Technically, she hasn't passed eighth grade, but since Washington is grades nine through twelve, I talked to the administration there. We agreed it would be best to promote her instead of returning her to a middle school environment."

My mother bopped her head up and down vigorously. The movement stirred up the smell of nicotine in her hair, and I sneezed. "She's an underachiever, just like her brother. I saw a show about this on *Primetime*. It's the kids these days. They just want everything handed to them."

Mr. Shing shook his head slowly and showed us out of the office.

# CHAPTER THREE

I MADE A new friend at Washington. My small class of five had been led to the cafeteria to learn the results of the PSAT that we'd taken. I didn't understand what the PSAT was. Our teacher, Ms. Reynolds, had explained it was a test for juniors but that as gifted kids we were being given the opportunity to take it early.

I sat on the hard bench and tried to follow what the woman at the front of the cafeteria was saying, but I could only pick out bits and pieces. A big girl with bleached-blond hair sat next to me. She tapped the tip of her pencil against the plastic cover of my Trapper Keeper, where my name was printed in black block letters. "Hey, smarty pants! That's you!"

"Huh?" I said.

She pointed her pencil at my score. "You're a National Merit Semifinalist!"

"What's that mean?" I asked.

"It means you're smart! Either that, or it's just more bullshit." She shrugged and flicked a thick blond lock from her eyes.

The bell rang, signaling the end of the school day. The girl turned to me again. "I'm Elizabeth, but everybody calls me Biz."

"Okay."

"You're supposed to tell me your name now, smarty pants." She stared at me.

"Oh, I'm Twilah."

"Ha! I knew that already. I read your name on your Trapper Keeper. Anyway, cool beans. Hella-cool beans. Do you like REM?"

"Yeah."

"Wanna come to my grandma's house and listen to some records?"

"Yeah."

"Well, let's go!"

That was the last I heard about the PSAT.

Biz and I became good friends. She had an amazing collection of records and tapes. Almost any band you'd hear on MTV's *120 Minutes* was represented among the vinyl she collected in milk crates she stored at her grandmother's house, where she lived.

We started skipping school together. We'd walk out the side door of the building after the first hour and walk the mile and a half to her grandma's house, where we'd sit and listen to punk rock and alternative music.

"The teachers think you're on drugs," Biz said one day.

"Huh?" I stared at the nest of Manic Panic pink hair piled on top of her head. Biz loved to dye her hair.

"The teachers think you're on drugs," she repeated, "because of how you walk out of class and sit in the hallway and how you sleep at your desk. I heard Mr. Morris talking to Ms. Lane. He said he knows you're stoned. They were trying to figure out which drugs you're on. Isn't that hilarious? You're one of the most straight-edge people I know! Like, you should wear an X on your hand you're so straight-edge."

I reflected on what Biz had said. I couldn't think of a response, so I settled for shaking my head.

Washington was the same as Sumner in terms of me not being

able to hear in the echoing classrooms. But my time at Sumner had been a respite from bullying. One day, as I was leaving my first-hour class, a boy I'd never seen before tripped me in the hallway. I threw my hands out in front of me and barely managed to keep my mouth from smacking against the floor. The boy yelled something I couldn't quite understand, and his pack of friends gathered in a circle around me and laughed.

"What the fuck?" I heard Biz's voice rise above the laughter. "What the fuck, man? What. The. Fuck?"

Next to Biz stood Derrick, a tall boy with a blue Mohawk. The bullies eyed him and backed off.

"Bunch of fuckin' losers." Derrick drew out the O and Z sounds in the word. "It's not your fault what your mom does."

"Huh?" I wondered what Mom had to do with me getting beat up.

"You know," Biz said. "Don't you recognize him?"

"Who?"

"That kid. He works at Taco John's with your mom," Biz answered. Mom had left McDonald's and was now working at the Taco John restaurant across the street from our school.

"So?" I said.

"He's fucking her. He's fucking your mom. Everybody knows! Dang, for somebody so smart, you sure are slow. Come on, let's go to my grandma's. I got the new Social Distortion album. Mike Ness is soooo hot! See ya later, Derrick!"

The next day, my first-hour teacher pulled me aside as I entered his class. "Vice Principal Wright wants to see you. Go to his office right now."

Mr. Wright was a stocky light-skinned black man who sat behind a black metal desk. "Hello, Twilah. I've called you in today because you've missed a lot of school. It appears you leave most days after first hour. What's going on?"

"I don't know." I stared at my hands.

"Twilah, it says here that you're Caucasian. Who told you that you're Caucasian?"

I pressed my eyebrows together. "My mom, I guess."

"Twilah, before we can become who we're destined to be, we need to know who we are." He paused. "Caucasian people have white skin because they ended up in the cold climates of Europe, far from original man, far from original civilization. You don't have white skin."

I stared at my light-brown hands.

"Original civilization is in Africa. That's the birthplace of the human race. The people who ended up white migrated away. Our ancestors stayed. They were kings and queens. They were artists and merchants and mothers and fathers in mighty empires. You have to understand this. You have to understand where you come from."

"Okay."

"Here, in the United States, the truth of the majesty of our ancestors has been hidden from us. It's been stolen from us. We have to take it back. It's our birthright, your birthright. With your intellect, you have the power to go anywhere and do anything. But to do that you have to go to school. You have to become educated. That's the way the game is set up right now. Okay?"

"Okay." I nodded.

"I hope you heard me today. Now, go back to class and fill your head with knowledge." He stood up and opened his door.

I walked out of the front door of the school and didn't stop walking until I reached the public library two and a half miles away. For most of the next month, instead of walking to school and sneaking out with Biz after first hour, I trekked to the library. I read every book they had on Africa and African empires.

"I could spit on you," Danny said. I looked up and saw his eyes peering down at me through the space between his swinging dreadlocks. "You're pathetic. You make me sick. I *should* spit on you."

I lowered my head back to my knees, where it had been before his voice had made me look at him. I studied the shades of grey in the cement beneath me. An ant scurried past.

"Are you just gonna sit there, you pitiful thing?"

I looked up again. Danny flicked his cigarette into the bushes and stalked into the building.

"He can be a dick, but he's super cute," said Biz. "Come on, let's go get some McDonald's."

I stood and followed Biz to her powder-blue Geo Prizm. I opened the passenger door and kicked aside some of the fast-food wrappers clustered on the floorboard.

"Oh my God, did you hear Andy on that last call? He upsold three Power Ranger videos. That's three dollars in commission on one call! He told me it was an old lady. He convinced her that her grandkids would disown her if she didn't buy them. He's so hilarious! Oh my God. I'm so in love with him," Biz gushed.

There were more empty Burger King bags on the dash. The clutter made me anxious. I rolled the bags up and forced them into the pocket of the door.

"What do you want?" Biz asked as we pulled up to the order box.

"Uh, a Quarter Pounder and a Sprite."

"Let's take this back to the breakroom and eat it. I want to see Andy again," Biz suggested.

"Alright."

I now lived with Biz, who had moved out of her grandma's house. Now we both lived with her mom, her sister, Renee, and her brother, Kevin. Mom had kicked me out of the house after I'd gone home and screamed at her about the allegation that she'd been fucking my classmate. Biz's mother had moved her family to a duplex in the middle-class suburb of Olathe. I'd changed schools once more. Despite not having passed ninth grade, I got promoted to tenth because in the Olathe school district, high school was grades ten through twelve. The classes at Olathe North were more interesting than the classes at our previous school in the inner city had been, so Biz had started attending rather than skipping. Since I had no one to hang out with away from school, and there was no library within walking distance of the duplex, I tagged along. But I continued my habit of walking out of classrooms whenever I felt overwhelmed, which was almost daily. I'd sit in a hallway or a bathroom until my mind cleared. I didn't pass tenth grade.

It was summertime now, and Biz and I were working at the Pizza Hut call center in the suburb of Overland Park. We were back in the breakroom. "Hey, like, my mom says she can't afford for you to stay with us anymore," she said before she took a bite out of her burger. "I'm sorry."

I stared at my fries. "Alright." I got up and walked to the phone that hung on the breakroom wall. I dialed my old phone number.

"Y'hello?" Mom's voice came across the line.

"Uh, Mom, I need to come home."

"Have you learned your lesson? I only let my kids leave and come back one time. Next time, you're out for good. I'm losing the house 'cause of Burt, so you're gonna have to wait a few weeks until I get set up at my boyfriend's place."

"Terry has his own place now?"

"No, hon. I met my soulmate. His name is George."

❧

Biz drove the Prizm through unfamiliar streets. "This is pretty fucking ghetto," she said as we pulled up in front of a small house. Many of the houses we'd passed had boards nailed across the windows.

"A cat just ran into the gutter!" I shrieked and pointed out the window.

"That wasn't a cat. That was a rat."

Biz pulled to the curb in front of the house, even though the gravel driveway was empty. My eyes fixed on the big orange dog that lay in the front yard. It was chained to a tree.

"There's a fuckin' toilet bowl in the yard," Biz said. I pulled my eyes from the dog. A mud-caked toilet bowl leaned against the porch.

"No shit," I murmured.

"No shit? How can you tell from here?" she asked.

We both started giggling.

# CHAPTER FOUR

OKAY, DOCTOR, WE'VE gotta skip ahead here. The things that ended up happening at that house, they changed me. I don't want to talk about it right now.

*That's fine. We can skip it. How'd you end up in college?*

Oh boy, how do I make this succinct? Well, the last high school I went to was Wyandotte. They put me in eleventh grade there. It was horrible. If I'd thought the ass beatings I'd gotten at Washington were bad, Wyandotte was worse. My mom signed a sheet giving her permission for me to drop out since I wasn't eighteen yet. I'd kept moving around. I bounced from place to place. I'd moved out of her and George's house and stayed for a while with a girl named Jessie and her parents, who lived a couple of houses down from Mom and George.

Jessie helped me figure out the bus route to the GED testing center. As soon as I'd scrounged the money for the bus and the test itself, I'd gone and taken the GED. So, in the spring of 1993, when I was supposed to have been a senior in high school, I started classes at

Kansas City Kansas Community College. Mom was eager to help me fill out the financial aid paperwork. It meant I was doing something that would keep me from ever moving back in with her again.

So, anyway, I met this guy through Biz. Biz was popular. She called herself a social butterfly. She knew kids from all over the city. I have no idea how or where she met them. I mean, she knew kids all the way from the far southern suburbs of Kansas to the far eastern suburbs of Missouri. Anyway, she introduced me to this guy named Matt. We met in the summer of '93. He'd just graduated from a high school in southern Johnson County, which is a wealthier area. He was getting ready to go to the University of Kansas to study art. He was really quiet and really sweet. He was my first real boyfriend. When he moved to Lawrence to go to KU, I went with him.

When I saw the awesome stuff he was studying, art history and science and stuff like that, I applied to KU. Based on my GED score, ACT score, and grades from my two classes from KCKCC, I was accepted. Once I got into KU, I went to the campus clinic and asked for a hearing test. I couldn't understand what people were saying most of the time, but the audiologist told me my hearing was normal. I compensated for my inability to hear in large classrooms by reading my textbooks from cover to cover and by reading stacks of supplemental material at the library. College was awesome. The abundance of new information filled me with a joy I'd never experienced. When I was learning, it felt like I'd landed on Mount Meru. Like I'd gone to heaven.

"What are you doing tonight?" my neighbor asked as he arranged a set of jack-o'-lanterns on the air conditioner that jutted from the front of his apartment.

"Handing out candy."

"You're from KCK right?" he continued.

"Yeah."

"I didn't think they knew how to trick or treat in KCK."

"Yeah, we do."

He started yelling, "I was joking! It's such a bad part of town.

There's so much crime. It was a joke, dummy! I was joking!"

As soon as I'd moved to Lawrence, I'd realized that people were constantly making fun of where I was from. I'd forced myself to cloak my humiliation with a laugh. I'd detected a pattern. People became enraged if I didn't force myself to laugh after they'd told me I'd failed to understand they were joking.

I had a handful of new friends. They were people I'd gravitated toward because they were really smart and seemed to have their lives together. They didn't bullshit and half-step. They did things, and they made things happen.

But there was this fucked-up dynamic. I wanted to be like my friends, but in a lot of ways I just wasn't. Most of them came from amazing families. Their parents were high achievers too—professors, attorneys, and engineers. I was a peer age-wise, and I fit in fine as long as we focused on academics. But we were young, and sometimes the conversations digressed to things outside of school. That's when I felt like an alien dropped onto a hostile planet. My new friends would say the most outlandish things. They'd talk about living in the student ghetto, when, you know, I'd just come from the real ghetto, so I didn't appreciate the term. They'd call themselves poor, but they always had food and clothes. Their parents paid their rent. We were in a place where most people weren't violent, a place where we were safe and comfortable. But despite all that, my friends were complaining. The behaviors of the humans around me still made zero sense.

～❦～

"I'd like a pound of roast beef, please," said the tall woman with coal-black hair.

I leaned forward and strained to hear her over the sound of the meat slicer whirring behind me.

"I'm sorry. What was that?" I asked.

"I said I'd like a pound of roast beef," she yelled. "You need to pay attention!"

My face reddened as I reached into the deli case and carefully pulled a handful of slices from the pile. "Can I get you anything else?"

"Yes. I'd like a slice of cheese pizza and a medium drink. And I'll pay back here."

I couldn't hear what type of pizza she'd asked for, so I pointed my spatula at the pieces on display.

"Which one?" I asked.

She pointed to the piece she wanted. It had worked. I'd avoided being shouted at again.

"What are you mixed with?" she asked as I rang her up. The cash register was far enough from the deli noise that I could finally hear her.

"I'm Native," I said.

"Native? Really. What tribe? I'm Lakota. I go to Haskell."

"Uh, Cherokee."

"Cherokee. Uh-huh. I'm sure you are." She roughly pulled the receipt from my hand and walked away.

I knew it was a lie, but I didn't know what else to say. I knew by then that Mom's stories about our Cherokee and Black Irish heritage were bullshit. I'd stopped believing every single thing my mother said when hell had descended when I was thirteen. But there I was, brown for no reason, and I had to explain it somehow.

I headed to the bakery department to talk to Jasmine. The interaction with the Lakota woman had stirred up some thoughts I hoped Jasmine might be able to help me with. Jasmine was confident and proud of her heritage. She was in a black sorority whose members wore matching blue and white sweatshirts.

"I don't think I'm Native like my mom says. I think she's lying about who my dad is. I think my dad's black."

Jasmine threw up her hands and covered her face. "I don't want to hear it! That sounds like it's off Oprah or something." Her words came out loud and fast, and I took a step back. Her reaction taught me to never speak of it again.

⁓⋖⋗⁓

"Hey, sis, it's Jeffrey," said the voice on the other end of the phone. "Hey, what's up?"

Jeffrey was the only person in my family I still spoke to, and we only talked once or twice a year.

"Mom's living out of her car. It's parked in the parking lot of that truck stop off Eighteenth Street," he said.

"No shit?"

"No shit, sis. I can't help her. I'm broke. I don't even know if I wanna help her after what she put us through."

"I know what you mean. I can't do anything either. I got a full ride this year, so I quit my job at the grocery store to work on a research project. I don't have any money."

"That's okay. I just thought you should know that's what's going on."

I hung up the phone and closed my eyes. I could envision the jeers and taunts that would rain down if I opened my mouth and asked someone to help me figure out what to do about my mom living in her car.

I took a handful of Tylenols and called my roommate at work. "Be careful when you come home. I'm going to be dead," I said.

An ambulance pulled up to the apartment complex. Two young blond male EMTs put their hands under my arms and hefted me out of my apartment. I didn't say anything. I just pressed my eyes closed to block out the flashing lights on the ambulance, the sounds of the EMTs' voices, and the almost painful sensation of strange hands against my skin.

When I opened my eyes again, I was in a hospital lobby. One of the EMTs was talking to a security guard. The guard had a gun and a badge and stood like a soldier. He positioned his big body in front of a short nurse who angled the bed and pushed me down a hallway. She wheeled me into a big room and planted me between two thin curtains. Then she turned and walked away.

A tall, pale man in light-green scrubs approached the foot of my bed.

"You're going to have to stay here for a few days," he said. His arms were crossed as he stared down at me.

I struggled to protest through my tears. "I, I, I don't want to."

His eyes narrowed as he pushed a clipboard in my direction. "It's the law," he said. "Suicide attempts mean a mandatory observation hold. I need you to sign this voluntary commitment sheet."

"But, I don't want to stay. How's that voluntary?" I almost expected him to tell me I'd heard him wrong, that he hadn't said *voluntary*. Because what he'd said didn't make sense. *Voluntary* didn't mean forced under penalty of law.

He raised his voice in volume and lowered it in pitch. "If you don't do it voluntarily, we'll get the ambulance to take you to stay involuntarily in Osawatomie. Would you like that better?"

I sucked in a breath and wiped my tears with the back of my hand. If I had to live through this, I knew I couldn't afford another ambulance bill. Osawatomie was at least an hour away. I knew what the word *Osawatomie* meant. It meant the state mental hospital. It meant straitjacketed, raging crazies. The people who went there never got to leave. I signed the sheet.

In the psych unit, I smoked cigarettes in a small glass room. Outside the smoking room, a television roared. I sat in a corner, knees tucked into my chest, as far from the sound as possible.

Nothing much happened in the ward. Sometimes other smokers joined me. I didn't mind the Asian man who sat talking to himself. Another man, a short, stocky white guy with matted grey hair, kept trying to lure me into a conversation. "Nobody cares about God anymore," he'd declare each time I saw him.

I met once with a psychiatrist. He was a thin white man with thin mousy hair. He wore a white button-down shirt and silver-wire-framed glasses. He shuffled some papers and asked, "Why'd you try to kill yourself?"

"Um, I'm just overwhelmed. Things are just too much." I stared at my hands, which lay clasped in my lap.

"What's so overwhelming?"

"Everything!" I blurted. My eyes were pressed shut, and I could feel myself rocking back and forth.

"What's everything?"

I searched for words.

"Everything. I got upset because my friends and I, we're all graduating in the spring. My friends are all excited. Their families are all excited, and they're throwing them parties and stuff. And I'm just lost. Nobody's throwing me a party. I don't have parents who are coming to watch me graduate. I don't even know where I'm supposed to go on graduation day. It's like there's this secret information everybody else has, and I didn't get a security clearance. It's not just graduation. Life's always been like that." I could tell I was mumbling. I did that when I was overwhelmed. I felt the warm wetness of tears on my cheeks and opened my eyes.

"Look, you're what?" He glanced at his clipboard. "Almost twenty-five years old. It's about time you learn to do things for yourself instead of doing things for your parents. Lots of people go to college because of pressure from their parents, and everyone feels stressed by graduation. You're not unique," he scolded. "How are your relationships? Do you have a boyfriend?"

I hadn't meant any of what the psychiatrist seemed to think I'd meant. But he was clearly very angry with me. I had no idea how to begin to explain how profoundly he'd misunderstood everything I'd said; and I knew any attempt to do so would make him angrier. So, to avoid his wrath, I did what I always did in such situations: I allowed the misunderstanding to stand and focused my mental and verbal energies on trying to placate my conversation partner by simply answering his questions.

"Um, I broke up with my boyfriend a couple of weeks ago."

"Have you had boyfriends before that?"

"Yeah."

"When did those relationships end? What time of the year?"

"Um, my boyfriend before that—we broke up last winter. I haven't really had many boyfriends."

"When in winter? What month?"

"Um, December."

"How are your grades? What's your GPA?" He was nodding for some reason.

"Huh? Um, around 3.3 or something—"

"So, your functioning is fine. You just need to stop having exaggerated reactions to normal stressors." He kept nodding. "Go to the groups while you're here, and you'll learn better coping skills."

*Your functioning is fine.* I reflected his words back in my mind. I couldn't assert myself well enough to use the phone to order a pizza because if the person on the other end got a rude tone, I'd panic and freeze. I couldn't navigate the bus system without help. I didn't know how to cook anything that didn't go in the microwave. I'd only recently figured out how to manage my own checkbook. My boyfriend, Matt, had handled that for me before. But this man was a doctor. He knew about functioning. And he said my functioning was fine.

I followed his directions and went to the groups. I sat silently, watching the other patients cry over things I didn't quite understand because I couldn't follow all the sounds in the large room with poor acoustics.

"Don't you have anything to add to this conversation, Twilah?" the group leader would ask each time a session ended and I'd been the only patient who hadn't spoken.

My face felt hot as I sorted through her words. I opened my mouth and forced out some sounds. "Huh? Um, no."

"Speak up please. I can't hear you," she said.

I opened my mouth again, but no sound came out. Tears were on my cheeks. I rose from my seat and ran to my room, where I pressed my face into the pillow and cried.

I stopped going to groups and divided my time between the smoking room and my bed, where I'd sit and read. At mealtime, I'd eat alone in a corner.

"Twilah, come with me to my office please," the psychiatrist called from the door of my room. It'd been three days since I'd seen him. I thought maybe he'd forgotten about me, but I'd been too scared to ask where he'd gone. I didn't speak unless I was spoken to.

He closed his office door and spoke. "I'm going to discharge you from the unit. You have seasonal affective disorder. It's clear from your history. I'm one of the pioneering researchers of SAD.

I've published papers on it. During your interview, you told me each of your past romantic relationships had ended in December. That fits the pattern. You need to start on Prozac, and you'll see an improvement in your mood."

I stared at my hands and pulled some words together in my mind. After I could see the sentence, I tried it out. "Um, I'm really not comfortable taking a pill for my brain."

"Well, it's obvious you can't get through winter without help, and this pill is help. Some people experience an annual depression. Their brains don't have the right chemicals to get through the months when there's less light. It's science. It's a clear solution. You need to take it," he insisted.

I took a few more breaths and visualized the words I needed in order to respond. "Isn't it possible that there's, um, a range of personality diversity and mine's at the far end of that range? I'm not comfortable taking a brain drug just because I react to winter differently than some people." I blinked, surprised that the words had come out as I'd planned.

"No," he said with a sigh and a small half smile. "You have a disorder that will respond to medication, just like if you had a virus. This medication will improve your functioning. It would be foolish for you not to take it. Foolish. You'll be able to think more clearly and solve problems better."

I stared at my hands and considered what he'd said. The contradiction was clear. I took a breath and fought to find some words. "I'm already functioning well the majority of the time. You said so yourself. I just got stressed. If this drug increases my level of functioning, wouldn't that be like cheating? Like an athlete doping for enhanced performance?"

"Oh no, no, no. Of course not. It's nothing like that," he declared with another sigh and a shake of his head. "It's a treatment for a disorder, like a splint for a broken bone. You not wanting to take Prozac is very silly. You can't expect to feel better if you won't go along with the appropriate treatment protocol."

Shame rose up. What he was saying still didn't make sense,

but of course I was wrong. What had I been thinking speaking my mind to a doctor? An educated man who'd surely come from a good family. A published man. A man who didn't struggle to form every word like I did. I felt the heat of the tears that always came when my ability to defend myself with words moved beyond my reach. I took the prescription from his hand.

# CHAPTER FIVE

"I GOT THE job, Beezie!" I cheered. I ran my fingers through my Australian shepherd's tri-colored fur and kissed the top of her head. "We're gonna move out of this roach pit. But I've gotta go to training up in Wisconsin. Your sitter will take care of you, sweet baby."

I attached a leash to her collar and opened the front door. "Ooh! Look at the beautiful day, Beezie! Sunshine, sunshine," I cheered.

I slowed, and Abiza slowed with me. I pulled my stocking cap down to my eyebrows and watched the wind ruffle my dog's fur. I smiled as I reached down to pet her. "You're a good girl, Beezie."

It was 2003, and I'd gotten a job with Indemnity National Insurance. I was excited, because compared to anything I'd done before, the pay was incredible.

※

The acoustics in the training class were decent, so I could actually hear some of the presentation. My eyes focused on the whiteboard as Judy, the trainer, used a squeaky blue marker to highlight key points. I never spoke. It took all my energy to follow her speech while copying the words she created on the board.

At break time, I and the rest of the Kansas City group gathered for lunch. A woman from the Indianapolis group joined us. She lowered her voice and pointed toward a woman from Des Moines. Indianapolis asked, "See her?"

The KC folks nodded. "Yeah."

"See her earlobes?" Indianapolis asked. I watched my coworkers nod again.

"You know how she jumps in to answer all the questions? You see how her earlobes are long? I bet she's got Asperger's," Indianapolis declared.

I leaned in to listen as Indianapolis raised her voice. "It's high-functioning autism is what it is! They can be really smart, but they don't have any social skills. That's why she keeps answering all the questions. And they have really long earlobes. That's a sign right there!"

I'd never heard of Asperger's before. I wondered if it was like Down syndrome, where a certain set of facial characteristics corresponded to a medical condition.

Training ended, and I went back home. I knew my new coworkers thought I was weird, because they said so to my face. They teased about me how I talked; I guess I used big words a lot. But they didn't peg me as having Asperger's. Must be the normal earlobes, huh? Anyway, when my coworkers teased me, I just told myself to let it go. I'd had years of practice in swallowing shame.

Everything changed when I asked Indemnity National for a transfer from the Kansas City office to the Topeka office to shorten my commute. I still lived in Lawrence, because I didn't care for change. I didn't have any reason to think a transfer to another office could go so wrong.

On my first day in Topeka, my new manager didn't take me around and introduce me to the team. But I'd learned in Kansas City that was the right thing to do—go around and shake hands. I was uncomfortable with that sort of assertiveness, painfully uncomfortable really, but I knew I had to imitate what I'd learned was social protocol.

I walked the aisles with my hand held out in greeting, but most of my new teammates just stared at me. Some mumbled and turned away. Only two or three people shook my hand.

Weeks passed, and I still had no idea why people in Topeka were so much meaner than people in Kansas City. My coworkers never spoke to me. One day, I took a deep breath and tried to initiate a conversation.

"Did you see there's a new art exhibit over by the capital building?" I asked the woman who sat across from me at the breakroom table. I stared at the small silver cross that dangled from a thin chain around her neck.

"We don't do that artsy fartsy stuff around here," she replied before standing and walking away. A few days later, I overheard her talking to someone else.

"Kansas City's a cesspool."

"Yes, it is, with all that crime."

"No morals."

"Gangs. That's diversity for ya," Cross Lady finished before returning to her desk.

My cubical was attached to the cubical of a man I began to think of as Foghorn Bighorn. His gigantic voice was constantly bleating, "Yeah, you think the Chiefs are gonna do it this year? What about the Wildcats? Gotta watch out for Oklahoma! Big Red!"

I stood behind Bighorn as I waited to ask our supervisor a question.

"Hey, Doug," Bighorn boomed. "You ever see one of these tribal police reports? I got one from the Potawatomi reservation."

Doug looked up. "No, man, I haven't. What's it say? *How. Me see cars go boom?*" he teased.

Bighorn bent over laughing. "You're funny as hell, man."

I sucked in a breath and froze. As soon as I could exhale, I walked back to my desk. I pushed my tensed shoulders down and hammered out an email to Doug. I knew I'd never get past my first sentence if I confronted him verbally. If he responded with a rapid verbal counterstrike, I'd become confused and mute.

When I opened my email the next day, I saw that Doug had sent an apology for his statement. But my other coworkers continued with the racist chatter. My cheerful hellos were met with cold stares. I started to make mistakes. My evaluation scores plummeted from the rating of "excellent" I'd had in Kansas City to the "needs improvement" category.

I called Blue Cross and asked for a referral to a therapist. A few days later, I pressed a buzzer next to the name of the social worker the Blue Cross rep had given me. The door clicked open, and I walked up a short flight of stairs. At the top of the staircase stood a closed door and a sofa. I sat on the sofa and stared at the door. My fingers drummed against my thigh. I counted ceiling tiles and glanced at my watch.

It was now twenty minutes past my appointment time. I panicked. I turned over the question of whether I should get up and knock. Under any other conditions, I would've abandoned the appointment—just gotten up and left, but I needed help. I considered whether this might be a test. Perhaps the therapist was gauging my character by determining whether I'd knock on the door. I couldn't start out by failing. My stomach churned as I stood. I hit the door with two short raps of my knuckles. A voice yelled a garbled response, and I scurried back to the sofa.

A couple of more minutes passed before the door opened and a man and woman exited. A woman with shaggy gray hair peeked her head out after them and gestured with her hand for me to come in. I peered into the large room, taking in red brick walls and giant windows. I squinted as bright light shone in from the direction of the street, but I stopped my hand from lowering my sunglasses from my head to my face. I knew people didn't approve of wearing sunglasses indoors.

"Well, you don't have to stand there. You can come on in and have a seat. I'm Jane. You were referred by Blue Cross?"

"Um, yeah," I said as I lowered myself into an armchair. It was deep. I sat at the edge so my feet could touch the floor.

"Okay. Why are you coming for therapy?" I read all the writing on the master's of social work degree that hung framed on the wall behind her before closing my eyes. She'd graduated in 1974, one year before I was born.

"Um, I'm having problems at work. I have a good job, but my coworkers hate me."

"We can work on that. Anything else?"

"Um, I think some things from my childhood might be affecting me too." I opened my eyes enough to peek at Jane, then I turned my gaze to my lap.

"No, I don't think so."

I wondered if I'd heard her right.

She went on, "You look like the daughter of an attorney and an accountant. You're really pretty. I don't think you had a bad childhood."

I felt heat spreading up my neck. It had taken so much effort to speak the word *childhood*. *I think some things from my childhood might be affecting me*. I'd visualized the words over and over for days until I'd become comfortable with them. But as soon as they'd left my mouth, Jane had shut me down. I tried to find new words with which to respond. None appeared, so I waited for Jane to speak.

"We'll work on your job situation, and you'll be fine." When I glanced up from my lap, I saw her lips were pressed together and turned up at the corners.

"Oh, okay," I said. I guessed that was how therapy with Jane worked.

The next week, I revealed my dilemma. "I can't talk in groups. I've never been able to talk in groups. We had another meeting today, and I wanted to contribute, but I couldn't."

"Well, you should understand by now that there's nothing to be afraid of. You're really pretty. There's no reason for you to have all these self-esteem problems. Just speak," she said as she crossed her arms.

"I try to, but by the time I figure out what to say, someone else is already talking—"

"Just be confident and speak! You're plenty intelligent, and you're so pretty. You just have to have confidence. That's all there is to it. Everybody can talk!" She frowned.

"I try, but—"

"Don't *try*. Do!" Her words had begun to sound clipped.

"But I can't. I just can't—," I declared as tears rose up.

"Well, with that attitude, you never will."

The tears ran down my cheeks in a hot stream. If speaking in groups was as simple as Jane said, why was I almost thirty years old and still unable to do it? I'd read books on assertiveness and still couldn't always speak when I needed to. My sobs began to catch in my throat.

"Hopefully we can work on something else next week. You've had plenty of time to figure this out," Jane sighed. I glanced up and saw her eyes were slit and her lips were slightly puckered.

I lifted my backpack from the floor and hefted it onto my shoulder. I wiped my tears with the back of my sleeve and descended the stairs.

With each session, Jane seemed to become angrier and more impatient. "I had to ask to change desks because this guy Bighorn, er, Larry is really loud. I can't think over his voice. Now I'm sitting next to this woman named Cammie, and she's loud too. She shrieks into the phone, 'This is Cam-eeeee!' She stands by my desk and talks about weird things."

"What does she say that's so weird?" Jane asked.

"Stuff like, 'Billy Bubbles picked me up in his Ford F-350 turbo diesel, and we went to a movie. He's a cattle dealer in El Dorado. He's gonna get his daddy's ranch one day.' I don't know what I'm supposed to say when she tells me stuff like that."

"What did you do when she said that?"

"Um, I wondered where El Dorado is. I wrote *El Dorado* in all caps on my notepad to remind myself to look it up. Cammie just stood there staring at me, so then I said, 'Oh, that's nice. He sounds like a good guy.' But that seemed to make her mad. Now, she's doing more weird stuff. Every day right before five o' clock, she changes into her gym clothes and walks around the office in her sports bra."

"Just ignore her," said Jane. "I don't see why this is such a big deal to you."

"It's 'cause she hates me, and all her friends hate me, and all her friends are all my other coworkers, and they all hate me, and I hate going to work there, but I have to pay my rent and my student loans." The words poured from my mouth.

"I'm sure you're imagining all that hate. Stop making such a big deal out of this, and you'll be fine."

I tried to do as Jane instructed, but Cammie's behavior became more bizarre. The next day, she approached my desk.

"You're pretty muscular for a girl," she said with a small laugh as she stared at my biceps. "What do you do at the gym?"

"Uh, I just run on the treadmill on odd days and lift weights on even ones."

"Do you have a personal trainer?"

"I did in the beginning, and I do every now and again when I need a new weight routine. So, off and on, I guess."

"Is he cute? Do you think he makes a lot of money?" she asked.

"Uh, I don't know." Cammie had begun to glare at me again. Then she pranced away to flash her boobs at Bighorn.

I described the situation to Jane.

"I told you to just ignore her. You make way too big a deal out of things," she repeated. Something about the way she said it made me think she might be bored. She was definitely angry. But I had no idea how to figure out which people should be ignored and which should be engaged. I wanted to ask Jane how to tell the difference, but each question I asked seemed to make her angrier, so I stopped asking questions.

"Hi, is this Twilah?"

"Yeah." I waited for the person to tell me why they were calling.

"This is your brother Glen."

"Oh wow! Really? What's up?" I'd only spoken to Glen a handful of times in my life.

"I'm in Lawrence right now. I looked you up in the phonebook. Want to meet me at The Jazzhaus tonight?"

Over pints of Boulevard Wheat, Glen brought me up to date on his life. "I've got a daughter. We live outside of Wichita. But the most important person in my life is Jesus Christ. Do you know Jesus?"

"Not personally. But I've read a lot about world religions."

Glen treated me to an hour-long monologue on Jesus.

"We should get together with Jeffrey and go talk to Mom," he said. "She needs to understand how her life choices have hurt us spiritually."

"Uh, okay," I agreed.

Our mother had found a new boyfriend, an alcoholic, cross-dressing aerospace engineer. He'd moved her out of the truck-stop parking lot and into his suburban home. My brothers and I met at the house, which was north of the Missouri River in Kansas City. I followed as Glen stepped onto the porch and knocked on the door. After a moment, the door eased open. A grey-haired woman stood in the entryway. I fixed my eyes on the cane she leaned against. It was painted hot pink and wrapped in silver tinsel.

"Yes?" she asked. I stood on my toes and peered over Glen's shoulder. I hadn't seen her in years. I could smell the cigarette smoke coming off her skin from several feet away.

"Hi, ma'am," said Glen. "I'm selling magazines. Today I'm offering—"

"No, sorry, hon. I can't buy anything. I'm on a fixed income," she said in a shaky voice.

"Mom," he continued, "I'm your son Glen."

"Oh my God." Her eyes grew large as she reached out to embrace him. "I didn't even recognize you."

She looked over his shoulder.

"Oh my God, all my kids. Come in. Come in." She stepped back into a cluttered entryway, and we moved forward into the house. The stench of stale cigarette smoke caught in my throat. It was chased by a musty smell that got stronger as we followed her deeper into the house. She turned down the volume on a television before pulling herself onto a bed and waving at a corner.

"There's folding chairs over there. I'm so sick anymore, I just stay in bed," she said in her odd syntax. We each unfolded a chair and sat. She lit a cigarette and launched into a point-by-point guide to her maladies.

"A couple of years ago, my head blew up. Blew up!" She threw apart her hands for emphasis, and cigarette ash spilled to the floor. "And look at my gut! It's like I'm pregnant again. But I'm not. I had my tubes tied after Jeffrey. No, don't you say it. It's probably gangrene, I already know. Saw that on a show the other day. Gangrene is—"

"Mom," Glen interrupted. "We're here to talk to you about some important stuff. I'm up from Wichita, and I'm not going to be in town long. Can we talk?"

She swung her eyes from the television she'd been watching as she'd listed her ailments. She regarded Glen. "Well, sure, honey."

"First, I think there's something you need to clear up with Twilah." I scooted to the edge of my chair. I hadn't expected him to be so direct, for us to get to the point so quickly.

"Okaaaay. I don't know what you're talking about, Glen."

He kept his eyes pointed at her. "Oh, I think you do know. I think it's past time you tell Twilah who her real father is."

"I just never knew when it'd be the right time," she started with a small sniff. I glanced up and saw that her blue eyes were sunken into wrinkled sockets.

"Twilah, your biological father is a man I used to work with when I did factory work. We were on the company bowling team together. His name is Claude."

"And he's black, right?" interjected Glen.

"Yes, he's black." The words rushed from her mouth. The sniffle in her tone was gone. She was beyond confession mode. She was in the familiar territory of manipulation mode. "But that doesn't matter. Your real dad is Burt. He treated you like his own. He always treated you all the same."

I conjured up memories of the rare weekends when he'd been home throughout my childhood. He'd been a large, vaguely sad and silent lump fixed to the Laz-Z-Boy in front of the television.

Whenever Burt had been home, the TV had been tuned to *Hee Haw* or the *Grand Ole Opry*. He'd looked a lot like Don Williams whenever he'd worn his cowboy hat.

Mom's words were true. Burt had treated us all the same. He'd treated us as identical distractions from the escape the television had offered him.

I didn't realize I was crying until I tasted the salt on my lip as I bit it. I'd been sitting with my eyes clamped shut since her revelation. I opened them and adjusted a contact lens that had gone askew.

"Wh-wh-why didn't you tell me sooner?" I asked.

"Because it was never the right time. And I didn't think it mattered. It *doesn't* matter. You have a dad. You have Burt."

I don't remember what else was said while my brothers and I sat in that dank and smoky room. I cried tears of pain and rage, dazed by the extent of her obliviousness to my suffering. I don't know how much time passed before one of my brothers took my arm and told me it was time to leave.

After that meeting, I'd gone home and tried to kill myself again. My recognition that truth, trust, and identity were all so capricious had torn a hole into the foundation I'd believed I needed to exist. So, I spent another week in the psych ward at Lawrence Memorial. I left with another bottle of Prozac that I tried to refuse but had been bullied into accepting by the psychiatrist who held the keys to my freedom in the power of his documentation.

―❧―

I watched the red Pontiac pull to the shoulder of the road. "Hey, beautiful," the man called as he eased the car into park. I froze, unsure of what to do.

The man exited the car and walked toward us. "Beautiful dog too. This is my lucky day, meeting you two gorgeous ladies." He reached down and patted Abiza's head. Abiza licked his hand. *He must be okay*, I thought. Everyone said dogs had a sixth sense about people.

"You live around here?" he asked.

"Yeah, down the street."

"Let's go back to your place," he said. I liked his smile.

"Okay."

❦

"Tell me about your relationships. Do you have a boyfriend?" asked Jane.

"Well, I broke up with a guy a few months ago because he was a convict who wouldn't stop breaking the law." I watched as Jane narrowed her eyes and shook her head at me.

I'd come to think of the man in the Pontiac as The Demon. I'd tried for four months to make the relationship work. I'd tried so hard because I'd thought I could learn the guiding principles of blackness by having a black boyfriend. I'd never told Jane the story of my mother and her gigantic lie. Jane had made it clear from the beginning that my childhood had been fine, and Jasmine had said it was a story that belonged on Oprah. So, I'd seen no point in bringing it up. No one wanted to hear it.

"You sure like drama, don't you?" Jane asked.

"Huh?" I'd wanted to say no, because that was the truth, but I tensed with fear at the thought of contradicting her. She had power, and she understood people. She smelled the badness inside me and would chop me to bits with her words if I challenged her interpretation of my actions.

At my next appointment, I sat down with a smile.

"You look happier today. What's going on?" she asked.

"I met a guy at the gym. We're going out this Friday," I said.

"Really? When did he get out of prison?"

I paused, hoping I'd heard her wrong. After several minutes of her silent stare, I had to accept I'd heard her correctly. My face fell, and tears welled up.

But I had no one else to talk to, so I kept going back.

❦

"I'm still struggling at work. I don't understand how it is that I'm doing the same job I did in Kansas City, where everything was fine, but I do it in Topeka and I'm told my work is terrible," I said as I looked at the floor between us.

"You have to look at your actions and your choices. Your bad choices result in your unhappiness," she responded. Her words were saturated with disapproval.

As I reviewed her words, I felt empty and confused. I thought about my life choices. Did she mean it was bad for me to have gone to college? That made sense. If I hadn't gone to college, I wouldn't be miserable at a job that required a degree. Maybe it was a bad choice for me to try to succeed in a workplace where I clearly wasn't wanted. Maybe all of my choices were bad. Maybe I should've stayed in the ghetto where I'd come from. My breath caught as I considered that possibility. Fear and shame descended. I stopped scheduling appointments with Jane.

*I'm sorry that Jane didn't investigate whether there might be an underlying cause for your inability to speak in meetings.*

Huh? No, looking back it seems she thought I wasn't trying hard enough. That's why it was so hurtful. When I do anything, I do it 100 percent. To have her accuse me of not trying, when I was trying my best and still failing, was devastating. You know what I mean? It crushed me.

# CHAPTER SIX

IN 2006, A recruiter called me about a position with more pay. I resigned from Indemnity National and headed to Leader Insurance.

I'd gotten a little bit better at speaking in groups by then. I could speak if someone explicitly asked for my input, whereas before I'd just turn red and mutter that I didn't have anything to say. I still wasn't good at speaking on my own initiative because I could never figure out the right time to open my mouth and let the words come out.

One day, I was part of a committee that had assembled to make a decision about a contentious claim. I spun my head wildly as my coworkers offered opinions on how to proceed. No one asked for my input, so I kept my mouth shut. As we exited the branch manager's office, my supervisor pulled me aside.

"I swear, if you don't start talking, I'm going to smack you," he said. He was a tall man, and I took a step back to bring his looming body into perspective.

"I'm sorry," was all I could manage.

"What's going on with you? You're so hard to read," he continued.

"I don't know. Nothing. I'll try to start talking," I said before dipping my head and scurrying back to my desk.

I thought about the incident that evening as I ran my regular five miles around the park. Should I try again to find a therapist for my social anxiety? I didn't want to throw away money to be treated like shit. I was happy otherwise. Therapists always created new problems in addition to the ones I came to them with. I turned my mind away from the question and focused on the park around me.

"Hey, chippa monkey!" I blurted as a chipmunk crossed the path in front of me. I smiled. No, I didn't need therapy. I needed more time with the chipmunks.

---

I met a man online who worked in a hospital laboratory. I found his analytical thought processes captivating, and we shared a love of the outdoors. The only thing that made me apprehensive was that he had a nine-year-old daughter. I'd never cared for the company of children. But that negative turned into a positive when he'd reassured me he didn't want any more kids. Most men in the Midwest wanted a woman they could breed like a farm animal. It felt refreshing that he was different.

Let me tell you about something I figured out around this time, doc. I realized I have this problem with prosopagnosia, or face blindness, though I didn't know the term back then. When I connect intellectually with someone, I don't really see or remember what they look like. When I don't care about someone, or before I've connected with them, I see their features more. I'd already made an intellectual connection with Andrew before I met him, so when I finally saw him, his physical being was almost invisible to me. But I'll tell you because you might be wondering, Andrew is white.

Andrew and I spent much of our time together on the trails around our respective homes. We talked about fitness and health a lot.

"Who's your doctor?" he'd asked me early on.

"Um, I don't really have one. I used a walk-in clinic in Lawrence when I got sick. I haven't gone to a doctor in the two years since I moved back to KC. I'm healthy. I haven't had any reason to see a doctor."

"You don't get a yearly physical?"

"No." I paused. "Am I supposed to?"

"Well, yes!" He laughed. "You're supposed to get a physical every year, so your doctor has a record of your baseline. Then, if any of your metrics change, you have a better chance of stopping a disease before it's too late."

"Really? I'm not comfortable having somebody all up in my business with these 'metrics,' especially when there's nothing wrong with me." I paused to consider this foreign idea.

I thought back to the time my mother had taken me to the county health department. I'd left the appointment with bruises up and down my arms. "Your veins keep rolling!" the lady with the needle and tubes had exclaimed.

There'd been other times too. Like when I'd been eighteen years old and had awoken to an eye that had cemented shut.

Biz had driven me to the emergency room, and the doctor there had seemed vaguely angry. "You have pink eye that should've been treated days ago. This isn't something you wait on and then go to the emergency room for. You need to go to your regular doctor for things like this before they get to this point," he'd lectured. I remembered the hot rush of shame I'd felt as I'd sat silently wondering how a person went about acquiring a "regular doctor." He'd sent me away with a prescription for eye drops. A few weeks later, I received a bill for $700.

A few months after that, I'd been walking in a park when something had stung my foot. My lips had started to swell, and my chest had become tight. I'd torn my sandals from my turgid feet, which had felt like they were burning more from the inside than from contact with the sun-soaked pavement. I'd hobbled home and collapsed on the couch. I'd watched as the skin on my arms and legs had turned red and bumpy. I'd lain there for an hour drinking water and hoping I wouldn't die. I'd felt sick for days afterwards.

Then there'd been the time in 2001. I'd had trouble breathing after returning to Lawrence from a trip to Chicago. I still didn't have any health insurance. The emergency room doctor had put his stethoscope to my chest and declared that I had bronchitis. He'd sent me away with a prescription for an antibiotic. I'd filled the script and taken all the pills. Two weeks later, I still couldn't breathe. I'd gone to the walk-in clinic I'd used throughout college.

"Didn't the emergency room do a chest X-ray?" the old white-haired doctor asked.

"No," I answered.

"You have pneumonia," he proclaimed after reviewing the films. "You're going to need more antibiotics. Take this Z-Pak for ten days, and come see me again if it hasn't cleared up."

Ten days later, I still couldn't breathe, and the same doctor gave me another Z-Pak. I'd been so sick that I hadn't been able to stand and go the bathroom without help. I'd stayed at an ex-boyfriend's apartment for the duration of my illness. I'd missed so much work that I'd almost lost my apartment.

Then there'd been the kidney infection in 2003. I'd been at Indemnity National and had health insurance for the first time in my adult life. The emergency room doctor had sent me to see a specialist after that—a urologist. The urologist had looked at the images from the scan he'd ordered and exclaimed, "I've never seen this in real life. I've only seen it in textbooks. You have two ureters coming out of your right kidney. You should only have one. It's odd, but I don't think it'll affect your health. You may have a bit of reflux, but that's all."

I sorted through my thoughts and told Andrew about my health department experience.

"That's such bullshit. Veins don't roll," he informed me. "That's an incompetent phlebotomist blaming the patient for their inability to do their job."

"For real?" I'd been told many times after dozens of sticks that my veins had rolled. "What did you call it? A luh—bott—what?" I tried to arrange the letters of the unfamiliar word in my head as he spoke, but it wasn't adding up to anything I'd seen.

"A phlebotomist. That's basically an underpaid, usually undereducated person who draws blood."

"How do you spell that?"

"P-H-L-E-B-O-T-O-M-I-S-T."

I followed along, the letters stamping themselves out in my field of vision. I traced the shape of each letter with my finger on my thigh for good measure. It was how I remembered things.

"But you can draw blood, and you're not a phlebotomist—are you?"

"No, I'm not. Lots of medical staff can draw blood. Doctors, nurse practitioners, physician assistants, nurses—most anyone in health care *can* do it. But that's *all* a phlebotomist does. They can't run tests once the blood is drawn. That's what I do."

I nodded. This was all new to me. Aside from doctors and nurses, I had no idea what other health care roles there were or how people trained for those roles. I'd met a couple of nursing students in college. They'd seemed like pleasant, boring, and unambitious people. I'd met a few premed students too. They'd been trust fund kids pursuing the career of their parents' dreams.

"You should see one of the doctors in our system," Andrew insisted.

"You still haven't sold me on this idea of going to a doctor for these metrics. I'll think about it."

As time passed, I came to trust Andrew and his insights into health care. A few months into our relationship, I visited one of the doctors in the Suburban Health System. Appointments with Dr. Vite were brief and superficial. He'd put his stethoscope to my chest and ask me to breathe. Then he'd order a few blood tests. Andrew would draw the blood from my veins. The process was painless, and he always got me on the on the first stick.

Sometimes, I'd pee in a cup. I learned that my bloodwork was normal. I also learned that some of the time my pee showed a urinary tract infection, even though I had no symptoms. Alternately, I'd feel like I had a urinary tract infection, but my urinalysis would come up clean.

~~

"Let me show you how it works," said the man who'd come to install the cable in our new home. Neither Andrew nor I watched TV, but Andrew's daughter, Caitlyn, enjoyed a few shows.

"Okay."

"Sit down there on the couch." He waved toward the faux suede sofa.

I sat as he'd instructed, and he positioned himself next to me. His body pressed against mine. Then his hand was on my thigh. I froze. He raised the remote in his free hand and clicked the *on* button. His left hand gripped my leg more tightly.

"You've got over a hundred channels," he said as his hand inched up my leg.

"I think I'm gonna poop." The words flew out of my mouth.

Cable Guy's head reared back like a cobra's. He stood and headed for the door.

"The cable's on," I said when Andrew came home. "Could you handle any other installs we have?"

"Sure, honey. Did everything go okay?"

"Yeah, yeah, the cable's on. I just don't like dealing with service people."

It would be months before I told Andrew the truth of what had happened that day. I was afraid he'd become angry at me for not standing up for myself. Shame often overlaid my silence.

Months later, I stirred black beans into a bowl of diced tomatoes. I layered the mixture between tortillas and covered it in cheese. At around age thirty, I'd finally figured out how to cook simple dishes that didn't go in the microwave.

"This is good. Thank you," said Andrew as we ate.

"Yeah, this is good, Twilah. Thank you," seconded Caitlyn.

"You're welcome. I'm glad you like it." I smiled. A warm sense of accomplishment filled me.

"I'm not feeling well though," said Andrew. "I'm gonna go lie down. Caitlyn, will you help Twilah clean up, please?"

"Sure, Dad."

An hour later, I was steering the car down the road. "My God, honey, I don't know what's happening. I've never had chest pain like this."

Not long after, the emergency room doctor seemed equally concerned. "Do you have a history of heart trouble?" he asked.

"No, not really. And I'm fit. I cycle over a hundred miles a week."

The doctor took a breath as his eyes scanned the pages in his hand. "This is your X-ray report. Your heart looks fine, but the radiologist saw a mass in your left lung. It's probably nothing, considering your age and health. But you should follow up with a pulmonologist to be on the safe side."

The next week, Andrew visited Dr. Plerra, who ordered a bronchoscopy. The procedure meant a scope would be lowered into his airway.

"We couldn't get the scope to reach the mass, so we can't say for sure what it is. Do you smoke?" asked Dr. Plerra at the follow-up appointment.

"No. I used to, but we quit together this year," Andrew said with a nod in my direction.

"What do you do for a living?"

"I'm a clinical scientist. I test specimens," replied my fiancé.

"Do you use solvents and things to do that?"

"I use some materials that require a high level of care, but no solvents per se. And I always wear appropriate protective gear."

"What are your hobbies?"

"Cycling, scuba diving. I have a pilot's license, and I fly when I can afford to."

"Oh yeah?" exclaimed Dr. Plerra. "I just got back from diving the reefs in Belize. You been there?"

"No, not yet. The last dive I did was off Cozumel."

"Ah yeah! Cozumel's beautiful! I saw a tiger shark last time I dove there," Dr. Plerra gushed. After a few minutes of diving chitchat, Dr.

Plerra seemed to remember he was working.

"You don't do pottery or glass blowing? Model airplane assembly? Any kind of art?"

"No," Andrew replied.

"I'm gauging your exposure to toxins," the doctor explained. His voice was confident, his eyes intent.

When the interview concluded, Dr. Plerra regarded us. "Even for a former smoker, at thirty-seven, you'd be really young for lung cancer. But we couldn't reach the nodule, so even though it isn't likely to be cancer, it may be a good idea to look at it. Or you can wait, and we can monitor it and see if it grows. If it grows, then we can decide whether to take further action."

"What does taking a look at it consist of?" asked Andrew.

"A surgeon would perform a thoracotomy. They'd separate your ribs and go in through your back to reach the mass. They'd remove it, and a pathologist would biopsy it."

"I've seen thoracotomy patients. That's a very significant surgery."

"Yes, it's very invasive."

Dr. Plerra answered all of Andrew's questions. He didn't seem rushed. Questions formed and dissolved in my mind, but I couldn't speak them.

At home, we discussed the options Dr. Plerra had offered.

"What would you do?" Andrew asked. "You're the rational-choice theory person in this relationship."

"I don't know. This is one of those situations where the only way to make an informed decision is to take radical action that makes the concept of an informed decision a foregone conclusion," I said. "The only way to get information right away is to have the surgery."

I'd finally found a person I wanted as a partner, and his life might be in immediate danger. I loved his mind. I loved our conversations. I loved the little house we'd bought and the husky we'd adopted. I'd even started to like Caitlyn. She'd reach for my hand as we walked through the grocery store. Despite my hatred of being touched, I allowed her to hold it. She'd look at me with a big smile when I'd tell her we were going to a Build-A-Bear Workshop or the zoo whenever her dad worked a weekend shift.

Two weeks later, Andrew's sister and I sat in a waiting area at Suburban Hospital.

"What do you think's going on?" I asked Sue. A respiratory therapist who specialized in sleep, she too had worked in health care all of her adult life.

"I don't know. They said it would take around three hours to get in and out . . ." Her words tapered off.

I returned my gaze to the beadwork I'd brought to occupy my hands. I threaded the needle through another tiny bead. The pattern and repetition were calming.

I looked at the clock. It had been chock-chock-chocking on the wall for four and a half hours.

A man in a white coat walked through the door. His bright red tie seemed too cheery for the occasion. "Twilah? Sue?" he asked. We were the only people left in the waiting room. He gestured for us to move to a smaller adjacent room and closed the door behind us.

"The surgery went well," he said. I exhaled and blinked back a tear. "We got the mass. To get it all, we had to remove the entire left upper lobe of his lung. Pathology is analyzing it. Whatever it is, I'm confident we got it all."

"How is he now?" asked Sue.

"He's doing fine," replied the doctor with a smile and nod. "You should be able to see him tomorrow." Sue asked a few more questions, and the doctor calmly answered them all.

A biopsy revealed the mass had been cancer. But it hadn't been a lung cancer like the kind that's caused by tobacco. It had been a carcinoid tumor. I didn't understand the difference, but Andrew seemed to think it was important.

After a few days, he came home from the hospital. His illness and recovery, and the stress of our impending wedding, had given rise to a sense of fear and hopelessness I hadn't felt in years. Andrew and I had become engaged mere months before we'd found out about his cancer. I'd never been a conventionally feminine person, and wedding planning was far outside the scope of anything I'd ever been interested in. We had no savings left after the purchase of our home, the deductible for Andrew's surgery, and the many other bills for his cancer treatment. We'd both taken unpaid time off from work once our paid time off had been exhausted. That had drained our finances even more. We had no parents to help us with medical expenses or wedding planning.

Long-departed feelings of alienation and isolation came rushing back. I'd find myself in bed crying, unsure of how I'd gotten there. Unsure how I'd get up. Strange thoughts coursed through my mind. I began to consider whether things might be better if I died.

I recognized the thoughts as foreign and irrational. I offered my mind substitutes. I meditated on gratitude. I wanted to be there for my fiancé, his daughter, Caitlyn, and our dog, but a never-ending onslaught of intrusive, destructive feelings exterminated my best intentions.

# CHAPTER SEVEN

I PLACED MY hands on the check-in desk to steady myself. "I'm sick and sad, and, and, my stomach is killing me," I stammered. "Can someone help? I want to stay alive."

"It sounds like you've been dealing with a lot, and they have programs to help you through tough times upstairs," the ER doctor said after I explained that I'd started to feel overwhelmed while caring for my husband as he recovered from surgery.

"Upstairs?" I echoed.

"Yes. We have a dedicated psychiatric ward. The staff there will be able to help you."

"Okay," I murmured. A young woman in scrubs escorted me to a room on the eighth floor. I lay in my assigned bed and cried. Through my tears, I watched the people who came and went in the hallway beyond my door. After several hours, a woman in a white coat stepped into the room. My roommate sat on her bed as the doctor began her interrogation.

"Hello. My name is Dr. Pintalabios." I'd read the name on my hospital bracelet, and the spelling flashed through my head as she spoke.

"You are depressed, yes? Suicidal, yes? For how long?"

I squinted as I listened. Her heavy accent obscured her words.

"I'm sorry? What was that?" I asked.

Dr. Pintalabios raised her voice and spoke more quickly when I asked for repetition. "I said, *you are depressed?* What brings you here?"

"Um. Yeah. I can't stop crying. I got really stressed because my fiancé had a big surgery and we have a wedding coming up and I'm scared and I don't know what's going on and I'm overwhelmed and maybe I should die." Tears welled up as I tried to rein in my sentence.

"Have you been depressed like this before?" Dr. Pintalabios asked. I saw motion out of the corner of my eye. I'd been staring at the bedsheet I gripped in my hands, but I looked up as my roommate walked behind Dr. Pintalabios and exited the room.

"Huh? Have I been depressed before? Is that what you said?"

"Yes." Dr. Pintalabios stared at me.

"Um, yeah. A few years back—"

"Did you take medicine for it?" she interrupted.

"Uh, yeah. Prozac. But it made me feel sick and angry, so I stopped taking it."

"We'll try Paxil this time. How is your sleep?"

"Huh? Uh, my sleep? Um. It's hard to sleep."

"You need Seroquel for sleep then, maybe trazadone." She made some notes on her legal pad. "Go to groups. Groups will help you. I see you again tomorrow or the day after, okay?"

The doctor turned and left the room.

I sat on my bed for a few minutes after she'd left, then ventured into the hallway to explore my surroundings. I peered through small windows that were set into double doors. I saw chairs arranged in a circle. People seated in the chairs were talking. I scurried away. I didn't want anyone to see me and make me sit in the circle. The thought of joining a group made my stomach bind up in knots.

The next day, a man with a thick shock of white hair came to my room. "I'm Mike. I'm your social worker. Follow me." I followed him to a small room, and he closed the door behind us.

"The emergency room report says you feel stressed because your fiancé got sick and your wedding is coming up."

"Huh? Um, yeah."

"You'll be okay. You see, even good events like weddings can trigger stress. When you combine them with other stressful events, like your fiancé's illness, you can expect to feel depressed. It's perfectly normal."

I tried to follow his speech as he explained how my depression would pass. His voice was soft. I lost track of his words and closed my eyes. After I stopped nodding, he wrapped up his presentation.

"Take the medications Dr. Pintalabios prescribes and focus on how this stressful period in your life is just temporary. And go to the groups. You should join the other patients for meals too. I've heard that you sit alone in your room all day."

"Huh? Um. Okay. I'll try," I lied. The thought of joining other patients for meals or groups sent an electric wave of panic through me.

After he released me, I inspected the ward again. It had three patient lounges, each with a blaring television. I rushed back to my room to avoid the cacophony.

"You need to stop isolating. Didn't your social worker just tell you that?" asked the nurse who had come to take my vitals.

"What?"

"You need to come out of your room. Isolation makes depression worse," she insisted. "You're not going to get better by isolating."

I absorbed her words but couldn't respond. I ignored her advice and stayed in my room.

Five days later, Dr. Pintalabios was back. "You're better now. You can go home. Keep taking your medicine, or you'll end up back here. You don't want that, no? Don't stop taking your medicine this time."

When I returned to work, my supervisor strode over to my desk. "I see you're back. We need to talk. Meet me in the Dakota room at nine."

At nine, we sat side by side at a conference table. "We've decided not to move forward with your training. You won't be going to the management course in Michigan."

My eyes widened. "Whaa—"

"You're no longer a candidate for promotion, is what I'm saying. It has nothing to do with you going to the hospital. Nothing at all. We're just changing course with our goals and needs as a company," he added without taking a breath. "We're going to assign your team to Travis. He'll be going for leadership training; you'll be going back to the floor.

"You know, you really just have to pick yourself up and get over this. Shake it off. Pull yourself together. I've had problems with anxiety before and I pulled myself together, because that's what people have to do."

I felt tears at the corners of my eyes. I stood and walked from the room.

֎

Local Hospital had refused to release me until I could show I had a plan in place for outpatient therapy. I'd decided to continue seeing Mike, the therapist I'd seen in the hospital. I didn't trust my insurance company to recommend a therapist, and I didn't know how else to find one.

I kept seeing Dr. Pintalabios for medication for the same reasons I stayed with Mike. While I wasn't impressed by her arrogant demeanor or the skin-tight leather pants she sometimes wore to see patients, I thought she'd be adequate for monthly ten- or fifteen-minute medication checks. I conceded that maybe medication was a good option, or at least better than the only alternative I was aware of, which seemed to a complete breakdown every few years.

I drove to Mike's office every Tuesday after work. On my first visit, I arrived wearing pressed dress pants, low sling-back heels, and a button-down shirt.

"Is that your uniform?" Mike asked.

"Huh?" I paused and pushed my brows together. My job didn't require a uniform.

"Is that what you wear to work?" He'd rephrased the question.

"Yes."

He nodded. "Where do you work again?"

"Leader Insurance."

"I think their office used to be near my old office. Their employees were always coming over trying to recruit us. They complained about their jobs all the time. They all used to go outside to smoke."

That didn't sound like my office at all.

"I'm pretty sure it was Leader," he continued. "They all hated it there."

I didn't hate it there. I wondered whether he meant I was supposed to hate it. I tried to figure it out as he droned on about how horrible corporate America was.

At the next visit, Mike asked, "So, how are you and the other keepers of the capital doing at that Fortune 500 company of yours?"

"Huh? You mean my job? Uh, well, it started out good. I got good evaluations, and I got promoted to acting supervisor within a few months of getting hired. They assigned me a leadership mentor who coached me on how to be a manager. My mentor gave good reviews to my supervisor and the branch manager, and I was about to go through the company leadership program to become a permanent supervisor. They told me my aptitude for business was excellent, especially for someone who'd studied liberal arts—"

"Yeah, yeah, I get it. You're really good at business, and you're really amazing and supersmart. You can do anything. You're so special. I get it. Yeah, yeah." Mike had cut me off.

I felt my forehead crease. I'd never had the incredible effort I put into my work pay off before, so I thought it was worth mentioning in therapy. But I'd said something wrong, and I didn't understand what.

Despite the shame I felt every time Mike mocked me or my job, I kept going back. I was desperate not to die, so I returned every week. I hadn't made any new friends in the three years since I'd left Lawrence, so I had no one but Andrew and Mike to talk to.

Andrew came with me to my next appointment. After we all sat down, I opened my mouth to deliver a revelation.

"I've noticed that my depression is at its worst in the two weeks before my period. After my period starts I feel better." I spoke with my chin lowered.

I'd practiced saying the words for days. Presenting this topic of a female issue to an older man was beyond uncomfortable. I held my breath after the words exited my mouth.

"Why wouldn't you have had this problem before?" Mike asked.

"Uh, I don't know. Maybe because I didn't have a period much until recently."

"Uh-uh, that doesn't seem likely," Mike responded.

I didn't understand if it didn't seem likely that I hadn't had a period much before, or if it didn't seem likely that my period had such a profound effect on my mood and ability to function. Either way, Mike's response made me think it wasn't up for discussion, so I closed my mouth.

"I really do think her mood problems are linked to her hormones," Andrew insisted. "She's okay for half the month. Then in the week or two before her period, she gets more anxious and scared. Sometimes, she even sleeps in the closet or tries to sleep in the bathtub."

"I don't see a problem with her sleeping in the closet or the bathtub if that's where she's comfortable. I often tell my clients to relax with warm baths. That sounds like an acceptable coping mechanism," Mike said. "The key is not blowing these things out of proportion. Not every unusual thing about our lives deserves a psychiatric diagnosis."

I spent a lot of time formulating ways to bring up other concerns in therapy, but each time I spoke, Mike shut me down.

"I really hate this habit my fiancé has of calling me every day at work," I said at my next session.

"Why does he call you?" asked Mike.

"I'm not sure. When I answer, he says he's just calling to say hi. But why would he do that? It's so irritating. I want to say, 'Well then fucking hi' and hang up. I hate being interrupted."

"There you go turning something nice into something negative," Mike sighed.

"But, but, I'm at work. I'm trying to *concentrate*! What does he think has happened in the time between me leaving for work at six thirty a.m. and me sitting at my desk at noon? There's nothing to talk about. I'm fucking working." I exhaled.

"If it bothers you that much, then don't answer the phone."

"I try that, and he keeps calling until I answer. He says when I don't answer he gets worried. I'm about to call off the wedding because of this. I can't work with someone who keeps interrupting me."

Mike's shoulders lowered again with his sigh. "Have you talked to him about this?"

"Yes! He gets mad and says he's just being nice!"

"He *is* just being nice. You're the one turning it into a big issue." Mike was shaking his head.

I pushed back tears. It *was* a big issue. If I got interrupted by phone calls, I couldn't focus. If I couldn't focus, then I couldn't do the job I'd worked so hard to get. But Mike didn't want to hear it, so I dropped it. As the weeks passed, I brought up other concerns.

"I have nightmares about bugs crawling on me," I said one day.

"Your real problem is that you shouldn't focus on things like that. It's just a dream. It doesn't have any meaning. You need to focus on not letting yourself get worked up over all these little things, things like dreams that don't have any significance."

I thought back to my teens when I'd slept on floors, couches, and dirty mattresses. I'd dozed in dirty backrooms and on cement. Bugs had crawled over me throughout the night. I could visualize the redness on my skin. I could feel the burning pain after the spots on my skin had become infected. I opened my mouth to explain, but Mike was still talking.

He was saying something about the importance of focusing on the here and now, not blowing things out of proportion, not getting bent out of shape because of every little thing. I hung my head. Tears came but words wouldn't. Soon, I was coughing through my sobs. Choking. The session was over. I grabbed a tissue and pressed it under my eyes, stanching the flood like a bloody wound.

"Maybe you should talk to Dr. Pintalabios about upping your meds," Mike said as he walked me to the door.

At the next session, Mike announced that he would no longer see me. "You look fine. You have a job. Your relationship is fine. You don't need to see me anymore because there's nothing wrong with your functioning."

That's when I learned you could be fired from therapy.

Not long afterward, I put in a time-off request for our wedding and honeymoon. The branch manager had called me to his office and roared, "You've been in the hospital twice this year. Now you're telling me you're too sick to work, but you're well enough to go on a vacation?"

"I'm getting married. And I need a break," I tried to explain. "Maybe after I get away and relax, I can come back at 110 percent."

"Giving 110 percent shouldn't require a break. You get a paycheck for it. You get to say you *belong* to this company!" he shot back. I emailed my resignation the next day.

⁓

***You suspected a hormonal component as a factor in your mood as early as 2007?***

Yeah, and I'd realized my period had returned in 2006. It had disappeared in 2001; '01 is when I'd started running and seriously working out. My period had gone away because I'd been so lean, and it'd come back when I'd gained more body fat. But no one had heard of premenstrual dysphoric disorder in 2007. And as far as understanding the mechanisms behind PMDD—the very first National Institutes of Health study on that came out in January 2017, so there was zero scientific understanding at all of what I was dealing with.

# CHAPTER EIGHT

"I HATE SEROQUEL. It makes me feel like I have worms in my head. And the Paxil's making me fat," I said.

"You don't take these medicines, you won't get better. You want to get better? You do, yes? You take these medicines, you get better. Understand? Simple. Like for cold. You take medicine, you get better. I give you Trileptal now. Try something new, it will help," Dr. Pintalabios answered. I struggled to follow her words, to pull meaning from her choppy delivery and accented speech.

"Can we test my cortisol levels? I'm wondering if an adrenal problem might be behind my anxiety. I wonder about my adrenal system and my energy levels in general. I've always needed ten or more hours of sleep a night." I'd practiced my delivery, and the words came out smoothly.

"Who told you about cortisol? Who told you about adrenals?" She flung the words at me.

"I, I—"

She cut me off before I could respond.

"You would have hair on your face if you had cortisol problem!

You have no hair!"

I'd been shaving the hair off my face for years. But she'd overrun me with speech, so I couldn't respond.

After months on Paxil, my diet had mutated from nutrient rich to sugar laden and carbohydrate heavy. Instead of going for evening runs, I baked evening cakes.

I hadn't put myself through college to end up unemployed, so I sent out resumes between crying spells and suicide attempts. For half of each month, I was fine. But every two weeks, with the predictability of sunrise, my mood would plummet, and I'd want to die.

I'd taken courses on finance and investing while at Indemnity National, and I'd done pretty well in the stock market before the crash. I managed to get a new job at an investment firm. The trainer for my new position was a woman named Barbara. She'd stand at a whiteboard and write down key concepts as she spoke. Sometimes, she would turn without warning to the class and demand an answer to a question.

"Twilah, name a risk associated with a money market fund."

"Uh, uh, uh," I stammered. I could feel the heat on my face as I stared at my notes.

"Anyone else?" Barbara asked after I'd lapsed from stammering into silence.

"Inflation risk!" offered the young man to my right.

Inflation risk. I'd known the answer but hadn't been able to speak. I sucked in a breath and waited for the embarrassment to pass.

Then there were what they called icebreaker and team-building games. "You've seriously never seen *Saturday Night Live*? What do you mean you never watch movies? Do you live under a rock? Stop trying to be such a hipster!" I tried to laugh off the taunts, but with each coughing chuckle, I fought back tears.

After six miserable weeks of training, I was put on the phone to assist customers. My coworkers' voices swirled around me. My fingers tapped my thighs nonstop. The clamor surrounding me fueled my anxious digits. A tone sounded in my headset, signaling I had a call.

"Millennium Investments, how may I help you?" I answered.

"How much is UGHX up?" a woman asked with a pace and tone that suggested she might've been better off calling 9-1-1 to report a homicide.

"I'm sorry, which fund was that again please?" I asked.

"U like Umbrella! G like Go! H like Henry! X like X-Ray! Jesus Christ, pay attention!" she shouted in my ear.

"UGHX? And you want to know what about it?" I repeated.

"How. Much. Is. It. Up!" she yelled.

"Just a moment please. Let me check for you."

My brain churned. I couldn't process the question.

"Hello! Hello!? Anybody there? I'm in a hurry here!" she shouted during my pause.

I typed with a frenzy, but I'd become confused. My brain wouldn't, couldn't, find the answer.

"I'm still here. Bear with me, please. I'm trying to find the answer for you."

"Jesus Christ. I just want to know how much this fund is up. Can you get someone competent on the line? I'm a psychiatrist here in New York City, and I just had a patient try to kill herself on me. I don't have time for this!" she raged.

I tried to ignore her shouting, but my brain had shut off. I typed but couldn't find the information.

"I'm very sorry. I'm not finding the information you're requesting. May I ask you to hold for a moment while I ask for assistance?"

"Well, it isn't like I'm asking for anything difficult! I just want to know how much my fund is up! Yes, get someone who has a goddamned clue on the phone! I just had a patient try to kill herself on me. I've had it! Jesus Christ!"

I raised my hand to get the attention of a coworker or supervisor, but no one looked my way. I pushed the button that disconnected the call.

Tears fell on my cheeks. I stood up and raced to the bathroom, where I sat in a stall and cried. I felt my lunch pushing at the bottom of my throat.

I told my supervisor a fabricated story of a family emergency, then I stopped by the human resources desk and dropped off my badge. I navigated home with eyesight blurred by tears. Another job gone. More income lost.

Dr. Pintalabios's response was to offer another drug, Topamax. I took it a few times. Foreign rage and boundless misery invaded my mind each time I swallowed a pill. I canceled my follow-up appointment with her and threw away the drugs she'd been feeding me. She could take her noncompliance and shove it up her leather-clad ass.

Her office responded by sending me a stack of bills riddled with inaccurate treatment dates and erroneous charges. I left several messages with her staff about the billing issues. No one returned my calls, and eventually the bills stopped coming.

❦

**How'd you go from not being able to balance your own checkbook in your twenties to doing well in the stock market in your thirties?**

What, you don't think autistics can learn things too? Seriously. Think about it. Those are two very different things. Investing involves a mastery of somewhat sophisticated economic concepts and elaborate problem-solving—totally my skillset. It's about evaluating risk and reward and projecting those evaluations into the future. It involves analytics and pattern identification. Balancing a checkbook is empty math. Numbers need colors, like sound needs letters. I can't master things that are empty, like numbers without colors. I don't understand things without an explicit explanation of context. You don't get that yet?

❦

I hopped from job to job. Some lasted days, some lasted weeks, a few lasted months. Training at each was a struggle.

"I'm just not getting it. I feel so stupid. This job doesn't even require a degree, and I can't understand it," I'd complain to Andrew.

"It's like this for you every time you start a new job. Don't worry, you always figure it out," he'd assure me.

I tried again at a mortgage company. During my first week I sat with Avis, a veteran employee who pointed at the computer screen and talked nonstop. She'd abruptly change topics, moving from the work task at hand, to events at her church, and then on to office politics. I'd become confused by her chatter and click the wrong link. Avis would note my mistake and begin talking even more quickly. "No, not like that. Like this. No. Here, not there. You see! Easy! You still don't get it?"

I wanted to scream at her, "Shut up. Just shut up, and let me look at it. I'll figure it out if you shut your damned mouth." But I knew I'd be called an asshole if I did that. So, I just stopped responding. I became completely silent as I struggled to tune out her rambling explanations and focus on the screen.

At each job, there were one or more resident bullies. At Balls Home Loans, that bully was Gloria.

"What's this with these special loans for Native Americans? That's bullshit. I'm Irish. My people were oppressed too. I want a special loan!" Gloria railed.

That was the cue for the racists to gather round her cubicle and tell stories about how all of the advantages granted to Mexicans and Native Americans had left them with nothing. I could never follow the whole diatribe, but there were key phrases that were impossible to miss. They were repeated like rage mantras.

"My kids don't get free college!" "Nobody gave me a handout!" "Taxed to the breaking point!"

*The breaking point.* I laughed out loud. I pictured the complainant, a gigantic, fifty-something blonde sitting at her desk, her face glowing red as she stared at the TurboTax program on the screen in front of her. Her varicose veins strained and throbbed against her denim capris and wound down to her Croc-clad feet. The Tweety Bird on her T-shirt was stained with salsa that had dripped from her Taco Bell burrito. As she touched *return* upon making a final entry, the trumpeter in a mariachi band sounded a single note, and her torso snapped in half with a dull crack. Her body fell from her chair, and her head rolled across the floor. An orange cat sauntered over to lick at the greasy spot that had formed on the ground near where her head had finally come to a stop.

I covered my mouth to suppress my laughter.

"What's so funny over there? I know I'm hilarious, but dang," Gloria shouted.

Down went my head, and up went the Rachmaninoff. I chided myself for my cruel thoughts.

꩜

Daylight streamed through the window. My body felt heavy, like it was anchored to the mattress. My abdomen felt as if it was filled with razor-sharp rocks tumbling in a current. I pushed myself up with my elbows but couldn't rise from the bed. I lay back again and reflected on how good my life was. I hoped my reflections would help me find the strength and energy to get up and shower.

*You have a husband who loves you. You have a job, even if it sucks. You have three wonderful dogs who need you. You have food and shelter. What's the problem? Get up and get on with your life.* I pleaded with my brain and body to no avail. My body wanted me to die.

I drove myself to the emergency room of Local Hospital. I followed a woman with a clipboard to a tiny room across from the nurses' station. The nurses' shrill voices and laughter echoed painfully in my skull. Several of them had gathered around the large desk, drinking out of Styrofoam cups and chattering indecipherably. My sobs became heavier, and I buried my head under the thin blanket.

I heard footsteps and looked up. One of the nurses had come in. She made a note on her clipboard and turned to leave.

"Excuse me. Can I be moved to a quieter room? This noise is making me more stressed," I said. The act of speaking shot a wave of terror through my body.

"This is the only room we have," she replied as she turned to walk back out into the hallway.

"Wait! Then can you close the door? Noise really bothers me."

"No! We can't close the door on a suicide case!" She spun and walked away.

After what seemed like hours, another woman entered the room. "I'm the mental health intake tech," she said as she closed the door behind her. "I have a few questions for you."

"Okay."

"What medications are you taking?"

"Phentermine," I replied after a pause. All the noise had made me confused. It was hard to see the word in my head before I spoke it.

"What else?"

"That's all."

"Why are you taking phentermine?"

"I'm overweight." My body was covered by the blanket. "I wasn't able to lose weight with diet and exercise, so my doctor prescribed phentermine."

After I'd stopped the Pintalabios drug regimen, I'd tried to recover my healthy eating and exercise habits. But running hurt my knees and ankles as a heavier person. Dr. Vite knew about my depression and the stress our family had been through because of Andrew's cancer. He'd prescribed phentermine to help me whittle down the weight so I could start running again.

"I see you've been treated here before for major depressive disorder. It's clearly recurrent with you. You need to spend some time upstairs again," she said.

This time when I went upstairs, I was told to undress so that a body check could be performed. Two young female techs checked my skin for evidence of cuts or injuries. There were none.

Next, another young blonde began to interview me. One of the body checkers remained in the room with us.

"How long have you been depressed?" the blonde asked.

"Off and on for the last two years, so since around 2006."

"And how long have you been anxious?"

"I don't know. For maybe a couple of years?" I guessed.

"How long have you had an eating disorder?"

"Huh? I don't have an eating disorder."

The women exchanged glances.

"It says here you're taking phentermine," Blonde said. She seemed to outrank Brunette.

"Yes, I am."

"Why are you taking it?"

"Because I weigh 155 pounds, and a healthy weight for my height would be between 98 and 130 pounds."

More glances.

"You don't look overweight."

"Well, thank you, but I'd like to be a healthier size. When I was in better shape, I was happier."

Glances.

"Okay, we'll take you to your room now. You'll see a doctor tonight or tomorrow."

"Okay, thank you."

I went to the lounge and called Andrew. I struggled to ignore the racket from the television in the background and tearfully explained where I was.

"I just wanted to die again. I'm so sorry. I wish this would stop happening, but I thought this was the right place to come. But I'm confused. These ladies here, these staff ladies—they asked me how long I've had an eating disorder. I think maybe they asked that since I'm on phentermine. Then they looked all crazy when I said I don't have an eating disorder. I don't want them focusing on something I don't have instead of helping me with my depression."

"Idiots," Andrew declared. "I'll call Dr. Vite and have him send a fax that explains your prescription."

I hung up the phone and headed back to my room, where I remained until I was summoned to meet with my psychiatrist. Another mental health tech led me to an office. "I'm Dr. Gaandu," said the brown man with scant black hair who sat in a big leather chair. I could barely understand him. I'd heard accents like his before, but I hadn't heard them often.

"How is your mood?" he asked.

"Um, I'm really depressed. This happens every month. I start—"

"I got this fax from your primary care doctor. It says he prescribed you phentermine for weight loss. I think it's very interesting you went to such lengths to hide your eating disorder. I don't know what you're so worried about. We don't even treat eating disorders here."

It took me a moment to process what he'd said. "What? I don't have an eating disorder. That's why I had Dr. Vite fax the letter—"

"Don't you think someone with an eating disorder would go to exactly that length to hide it?"

I lapsed into the choking tears again. After I sat sobbing for several minutes, Dr. Gaandu told me to go back to my room.

Dr. Gaandu prescribed Trileptal. After two days on Trileptal, my stomach was churning and I was more determined to die than I'd been when I'd checked in. I lied and told the staff I was feeling more stable, because I wanted to go home, where I could kill myself in peace.

*Could you see why Dr. Gaandu might have thought you had an eating disorder?*

Well, I can see that now. But do you see how absurd this is? If I'd had a problem with food, it would have been a binge-eating disorder. And I'd never had that problem before I was given the freaking Paxil!

# CHAPTER NINE

THOSE YEARS, 2008 through 2010, are a blur really. PMDD hell. I tried around ten jobs during that that time. Most were shitty, low-paid jobs that didn't require much education and also didn't require any intellectual effort from me. They never lasted more than a couple of months.

The less education a job requires, the more racists you'll find there. So, there was plenty of racism at these shitty jobs, and that stressed me out. Sometimes, I'd quit over that. Or I'd quit when I had a bad PMDD week and couldn't get out of bed.

I'd been having a lot of cramping with my periods, so I visited an obstetrician-gynecologist. This doctor believed me when I told him my depression correlated precisely with my menstrual cycle. He suggested I try a birth control pill to help with my mood and my cramps.

That added up to a daily cocktail of birth control, an antidepressant that changed every few months, a benzodiazepine, and the antipsychotic Abilify, which my new psychiatrist, Dr.

Boatbill, called a booster. With all that in my system, I seized a lull between suicide attempts and got another job.

Training at Flatland Insurance was hell. Seven of us were crowded into a tiny closet of a training room. The trainer, Casey, had a raspy smoker's voice.

"Then ya click here. Click there. Click here. Click there. No, Twilah—there!"

It was my turn to work through a claim in front of the class. I stood awkwardly, trying to sort out what I was supposed to do. I tried to watch Casey's mouth, but she kept turning her back to me as she spoke to the rest of the class. I squeezed my hands into fists and took a breath. I didn't want the class to notice the dampness in my eyes as I forced back tears.

I knew that once I was out of the training room and on the floor with no one squawking at me, I'd be able to do the job. I understood the processes. I understood the laws. I just needed a desk where I could master the software on my own. I just couldn't perform in front of the class with Casey barking at me.

A week before training ended, she pulled me into a coaching room. "Ron isn't sure he wants to bring you onto the team," she said.

"What?" I asked as I reviewed her statement in my mind. Ron was the department manager.

"You haven't shown you're a team player. You never speak in class. You never speak in meetings. And you don't want to do the graduation skit." After a long pause, I realized she expected me to defend my behavior.

"I'm a team player. I like everyone just fine. I'm just not very good at talking in groups," I offered.

"Well, you'd better get good. He's on the fence with you. Your insurance experience is the only thing that's gotten you this far. I don't know how you made it with those companies. Here, we're expected to communicate." She offered a hard stare, and I shifted my eyes away.

On my lunch breaks, I'd sit in my car or alone at a restaurant. I only joined my coworkers for lunch when to do otherwise would have been rude beyond a reasonable doubt.

Ron allowed me to graduate from the training class. As I'd predicted, once I was at my own desk with my own workload, I excelled at my job.

❦

My alarm made a soft click and started to play frog pond sounds. It was five thirty a.m. I opened my eyes. Cramps in my abdomen paralyzed me. I couldn't sit up or bend my legs.

I lay flat and tried not to move. Ten minutes later, Andrew's alarm let loose a clamor of electronic beeping. "If you hit snooze on that fucking thing, I'm going to launch it through the window when it beeps again," I threatened. The mere clicking sound of my alarm clock would wake me—I didn't even have to wait for the nature sounds. But Andrew needed the equivalent of a marching band to rouse him.

"It's off, it's off! Relax!" He turned and looked at me. "Honey, are you okay?"

"No. My stomach hurts, and I want to die."

"Do you need me to stay home?"

"No. Because I can't stay home. I don't have any more points to spare."

Flatland Insurance had a point system that tabulated absences. Any unplanned absence of any duration, and for any reason, resulted in the accrual of points. Numbers of points corresponded with tiers. Tier one was a warning; tier two was a write-up; and tier three was termination. No exceptions except for a death in the family. I'd reached the far end of the second tier.

"They can cram their stupid points. If you're sick, you're staying home." He pulled me against his chest, where I cried for several minutes.

After he left for work, I showered, but my tears wouldn't stop. I dressed and watched the tears form small dark patches on my fresh shirt. *Dammit! Stop doing this. There's no reason to be crying,* I repeated to myself like a mantra. My rational assessment brought no raft to the ocean of my misery.

I picked up my phone. "Hi, um, yeah, I won't be in today. My brother died." I squinted my eyes closed as the lie passed through my lips. Seconds later, I pressed end and fell asleep.

When I returned to work, my coworkers surrounded me to offer their condolences. I hated myself for having told the story, but I couldn't back out now.

Weeks passed, and I managed to stay under the point threshold. I got promoted to a position where I rarely had to use the phone. Focusing on fewer tasks made me feel less stressed, but the PMDD persisted. Andrew had become scared to leave for work. He thought that any day he'd come home to discover my corpse.

---

In the emergency room of Local Hospital, he held my hand as I lay on a narrow bed. "Can my wife be moved to a quieter room please? Sound upsets her a lot," Andrew explained to the nurse.

The nurse moved me to another room at the end of the hall. I pressed my tearstained face into the pillow as I heard the doors slide closed near my feet. Without the hospital noise, my panic eased, but my sadness persisted.

This time my doctor was a tall man with dark-brown hair. His tie was a shade of taupe that matched the walls. In the quiet of the small office, he asked me questions no one else ever had.

"Hi, I'm Dr. Brown. I see that you've been here before. When did you first try to kill yourself?"

"First? Like my *very* first try?"

"Yes, your very first suicide attempt. When was it?"

I closed my eyes. "I tried to hang myself in my closet when I was about eight."

"Why did you do that?"

"The kids at school beat me up and teased me. I hardly had any friends. And I thought I was ugly. I hated myself. And my mom didn't care. Nobody cared." I watched him make some notes on a yellow legal pad.

"Do you have nightmares?"

He spoke slowly, but his accent was hard to understand. "I'm sorry, what was that?" I sniffed and pushed the words through my tears.

"Do you have nightmares?" His tone and pace hadn't changed. He didn't seem angered by my request for repetition.

"Yes. Yes, I do."

"Tell me about them."

"Oh my God, they're horrible. I see the cats, and their heads are twisted backward. I hear the dogs crying. I hear his yelling. Oh my God, he won't stop yelling. He doesn't have a speaking voice," I cried. The images flashed through my head. I started coughing.

"Who is he? Are these nightmares from real events?"

"Huh? Yes. These things really happened," I sputtered out the words. I grabbed a tissue from the desk and twisted it between my fingers.

"Who did these things? What happened?"

I took as deep a breath as I could. I tried to replace the horrible images with a visualization of the Buddha. I had to find some calm to tell this story without my head exploding.

"When I was sixteen, I ran out of places to stay. I had to move back in with my mother. She was living in a dangerous part of Kansas City—a very violent, crime-ridden part. I'd moved out of her house when I was thirteen. Anyway, she had this new man when I moved back in three years later. He beat the dogs with a chain. He broke the kittens' necks with his hands."

I grabbed more tissues and pressed them against my face.

"He was always yelling. All he could do was yell. And I didn't have a room to stay in. I just had a couch to lie on. I could never sleep. There was so much screaming, especially when there was sex, which was all the time. I couldn't block it out. I'd hear it. All the time I'd hear it. The sex and the screaming." My eyes were pressed shut. My visualization of Buddha had been replaced with an image of my sixteen-year-old self, rocking back and forth with my fingers pressed into my ears, shrieking and wailing to block out the sound.

"Those are terrible, terrible things," said Dr. Brown. "What else happened?"

"Well, I'd wanted to go to college. I had a couple of friends out here." I made a sweeping gesture with my hand meant to indicate the surrounding suburbs. "Those friends—they were planning to go to college. I wanted that too—college—but my grades had been bad for years. Abysmally bad. I'd skipped school a lot. I was a junior in high school then. I thought maybe it wasn't too late to get my grades up and get into college. I started hiding in the basement with my books, trying to study and do homework. I was scared to go upstairs where my stepdad was. I'd come home from school and stay down in the basement for as long as I could. I used the cat's litter box down there to go to the bathroom. I did anything to keep from having to go upstairs."

I choked again and grabbed more tissues. Dr. Brown didn't speak. He gently pushed the box of tissues toward me. It felt like now that I'd started, I couldn't stop. This doctor didn't interrupt me, so my words flowed out.

"I told my mom how I wanted to go to college, and that made her really mad." Memories of the conversation invaded my mind.

"Mom," I begged. "I want to go to college. My friends are getting ready to go to college—"

"*There you go, always trying to be better than the rest of us. Do you think we're made of money like your little Johnson County friends' parents are? I wanted to go to college once too. I gave up a voice scholarship to have you kids. And I didn't have to do that. You were an accident. I could have aborted you, but I didn't. I gave up everything to marry Burt and have you kids. I'd like to go back to school too you know. I wanna be a teacher for retarded kids!*"

More tears came, but I couldn't find a way to convey the scene to Dr. Brown. My thoughts shifted, and I settled for telling another part of the story.

"I hated this guy, my mom's new husband. His name was George, but I called him Java Man—not to his face, but in my mind and to my few friends. You know? The Pleistocene Era remains in Java that scientists once thought were the missing link in evolution? *That* Java man. Not evolved, is what I meant. He was a fucking caveman. A dopehead imbecile just like all the men my mom adored. He made decent money, but he always blew it on shit. Drugs, cigarettes, cable TV—just shit. I remember one day he had a handful of cash, like a wad of hundreds. He was all happy because one of those traveling carnivals was in town. He's was all lit—" Dr. Brown glanced up and I clarified my terminology.

"On drugs is what I mean. He was yelling at my brother Jeffrey and me to get in the car to go to the carnival." I paused to blow my nose. "I told him to his face that I thought he was an idiot for blowing money at a carnival when we had nothing. We were so fucking poor because of his hedonism. I'd decided by then that if he tried to hit me like he hit everyone else that I'd stab him to death in his sleep. I had it planned out if it came down to that. Anyway, I went off on him, telling him he was a moron for blowing money on all this crap. He'd started raging at me, telling me I needed to learn to have fun, that I was a fucked-up kid who hated to have fun. Because fun is all about drugs and cable TV and wasting time and money, I guess. I think the only reason he didn't attack me is because it would've made him miss time at his precious carnival."

I glanced up. Dr. Brown was still making notes on his legal pad. I kept talking.

"I knew that if I didn't go to the carnival I wouldn't eat that night. So, I went. It was horrible—loud and nasty smelling." I shook my head as I stared at my clenched hands in my lap.

"I wanted to leave that house. I needed to get away from this monster, this Java Man my mother had married. I didn't want to have to kill him and go to prison. But I couldn't leave. I had nowhere to go. I'd run out of friends to stay with, and nobody cared how horrible Java Man was. Java Man had been yelling and beating the dogs and beating my brother that day. And nobody would help me. I couldn't handle it."

My head rocked from side to side as I stared into my hands. I could picture Java Man—the frames of his lopsided glasses a tarnished silver with two parallel bars holding the lenses together. The little bits of food clinging to his rat's nest of a beard. I pressed my eyes closed.

"Did you tell anyone about this when it was happening?" Dr. Brown asked.

"Yeah, I called the police. It took me days to get up the nerve. I was so terrified of calling strangers on the phone. I'd finally called, and I'd stumbled telling the dispatcher about Java Man and his violence. I'd only gotten a few words out. The dispatcher interrupted me and started making fun of the way I talked. She was like, 'Um, um, so my stepdad, um, um, like, um, like, um, um, um. Call back when you speak English, honey.' And that was it. She hung up on me. That's when I decided to cut my wrists.

"I showed my mom what I'd done, and she got pissed. She screamed at me with her usual, 'Always causing me problems, just like Glen. Always trying to act better than the rest of us! Like your shit don't stink! Now this! Now you go and do this with your drama!'

"Anyway, on the night I cut my wrists, my mom drove me to KU Medical Center. The staff there patched me up, but nobody really talked to me. The next morning, my mom woke me up. She was angry again because she couldn't find the razor blade I'd used. She wanted it back because Java Man needed it to shave."

I saw motion and looked up again. Dr. Brown had lifted his eyes from his notes and was gazing back at me. It seemed this was the only part of the story that surprised him.

He returned his eyes to his notepad and said, "Go on."

"I hated living at Java Man's house, and I'd done a piss-poor job of dying. I was stuck. Java Man would have his coworkers over for poker games, and they'd all get high. They were always yelling *nigger this, nigger that*. If I had to walk past them to get through the house, they'd yell things like 'George, why do you have a nigger in your house?' I had to leave."

I looked back up to make sure the doctor hadn't left the room. No one had ever allowed me to speak of this. I wouldn't have been surprised if he'd up and left. But he was still there. He was looking up again and regarding me with his deep-brown eyes.

"Go on," he encouraged.

"Well, I managed to rent a house. I was working at Pizza Hut, but I was only making $4.25 an hour. That was the minimum wage back then. I'd dropped out of school. My younger brother moved out of the Java Man house too and into the rental house with me. I had to feed both of us and pay the rent.

"That's when I did some stuff. Bad stuff. Men paid me for sex. Old guys. Nasty guys." I noticed my tears were less intense now. Maybe I'd needed to get this off of my chest.

I looked up from my lap again. Dr. Brown was still in his chair. "These things weren't your fault," he said. "You aren't bad."

Of course they weren't my fault. I'd always thought it was bullshit when I read about kids blaming themselves for the bad things that happened to them. I never had. It was obvious to me that Mom and Java Man were the fuck-ups in the picture. But it felt good to hear it from someone else. Another human being had finally let me tell my story.

Dr. Brown continued to speak. "I think you have post-traumatic stress disorder. That's what's behind your anxiety. Lorazepam will help you get that under control. You should also meet with a therapist."

"Therapists don't listen."

"There are some who do," he assured me. Maybe he was right. He'd listened, after all, when no doctor before him ever had. Despite the horrors I'd just conveyed, I felt a sense of peace. I departed Dr. Brown's office without tears.

A few days later, Dr. Brown ordered my release. His parting gift was a prescription for Ativan and a new diagnostic acronym of PTSD.

*Did you try to reach out to anyone besides the police when you were living through the hell at Java Man's house?*

Yeah, I'd tried to tell a counselor at Wyandotte about it, but I couldn't speak very well. I'd started by saying, "My family hates me," and she'd cut me off. She'd said something like, "All teenagers go through that phase. Everybody's got problems. Nobody has a perfect family, and everyone has family problems. It's how you handle your problems that matters, and you don't handle your problems well at all."

I'd interpreted that as meaning that everyone else knew how to handle a stepfather who screamed instead of speaking and killed animals with his bare hands. It was my problem that I didn't handle the situation right. That's part of why I wanted to die. That's not the kind of world I thought I could live in.

# CHAPTER TEN

*RING!*

I looked at the caller ID and gave a big exhale.

"Yes?"

"Oh my God, I'm so busy, and Daniel's just sitting here reading his Bible. Work's stacking up. There are specimens all over the counter, and Daniel's just reading and ignoring patients. Are you there?"

"Yes," I breathed.

"Are you okay?"

"I'm working." I could barely force the sounds from between my clenched teeth.

"I can't stand it. I'm working my ass off, and he's ignoring patients," my husband repeated.

"He's probably rereading the passage about thou shalt make your coworkers do all the work while you read about Jesus and collect a paycheck." I tried to keep my voice low.

"I hoped you might care about my stress!" my husband shot back.

*Ring!*

"Yes?"

"Oh my God, Dumpie mislabeled a specimen again. Thank God, Quest caught it, but guess who had to talk the Quest tech through how to fix it—just like last time? I told her she'd messed up, and she went off on me like it was my fault. Now she's hiding in the X-ray room even though there aren't patients here for X-rays, and I'm out here alone surrounded by specimens."

"Why don't you tell Donna about Dumpie? Tell Donna she's hiding out and refusing to work." Donna was the office manager.

"I was going to, but Donna's in the breakroom talking to a drug rep about her new Range Rover."

I didn't speak. I let the words from the earpiece swirl around in my head until Andrew realized I was no longer responding.

"Fine! Sorry to bother you! I thought you'd care about how stressed I am." His words came quick and angry. I hung up the phone.

I looked up and saw Ron heading up the aisle in my direction. He stood at my desk and further distracted me with pointless small talk for several more minutes. Then I saw the caller ID flashing from the corner of my eye. Andrew was calling back. I let it roll to voicemail. Finally, Ron walked away. I returned my attention to the task on my computer screen and took another breath.

"Team! We need to stop accepting personal calls at work," Ron announced at our next meeting. My face reddened as he looked in my direction.

That night, I relayed the announcement to my husband. "You know our department head, Ron? He doesn't want us taking personal phone calls at work anymore."

"What an asshole! What if I need to get in touch with you?"

"I'm sure it's fine if you need to get in touch with me in an emergency. He just doesn't want it to be a regular thing."

"What an ass," Andrew complained.

༄

Andrew drove us to see my mother in the public housing complex she'd moved into after her breakup from her alcoholic engineer boyfriend in the Northland. I scanned the directory to find the code for her apartment and rang the buzzer.

"Yeah?" A raspy voice came over the intercom.

"Uh, hey, Mom, it's me, Twilah. I'm here with my husband." I looked at the camera aiming down at me. "We'd like to visit with you."

"Is it gonna be pleasant? When you and your brothers came at me up north, it wasn't pleasant."

"I'll do my best to be pleasant."

I heard a loud buzz and the pop of an electronic lock. "I'm up here in 620. There's an elevator."

Andrew and I stepped into a lobby. There was a reception area, but the glass windows were closed. I saw a woman shuffling around behind them. Two clipboards sat atop a folding table. I paused.

"Visitors gotta sign in!" Shouted a voice from somewhere behind me.

Andrew and I signed our names on a sheet held in the jaws of one of the clipboards. Several old black ladies in wheelchairs shouted out greetings.

"Hi! Who you here to see, honey?" yelled a woman with a small salt-and-pepper Afro.

"I'm sorry?"

"Who you here to see, honey?" she repeated.

"My mom—Mrs. Davenport," I answered. Mom had kept Java Man's last name. It had floated out of my mouth before I realized I probably shouldn't have announced my business to this stranger.

"Oh, you tell your mama Ethel says hi," she yelled back.

I smiled and said, "Okay." I looked around for the elevator. Andrew stayed close to me. His body language was alternating between military-reconnaissance mode and look-natural mode. Reconnaissance was winning. I chuckled to myself.

We got on the elevator. "What's so funny?" he asked.

"Oh, just your demeanor. I bet Ethel's already on the phone warning that there's a detective in the building."

"You think?"

"Yeah, you don't quite fit in." I looked at my husband. He'd dressed in a blue pullover and jeans. But his erect posture, kempt hair, and clear pink complexion marked him as an outsider.

The elevator chimed, and we exited onto the sixth floor. My nostrils filled with the smells of cigarette smoke, sweat, fried meat, and onions. I knocked on the door of 620, which was covered in orange NASCAR decor.

An old woman opened the door. Her white hair was cropped so close I could see her grey scalp. She wore a thigh-length lavender nightgown and cotton-candy pink slippers. She leaned against a walker.

"Come on in." She waved us into a smoke-filled room. Pictures of wolves and touristy Native American art covered every piece of wall space that wasn't occupied by NASCAR prints. Stacks of boxes rose from the floor and all but one chair, into which Mom descended.

"Oh, just clear some of that stuff off the couch there and you can sit down." She waved toward a pile. I didn't want to touch anything. But I'd come for information, and it might take a while. I cleared a small space for Andrew and me to sit.

"It's good seein' you, hon. I hope this is better than last time when you and your brothers came at me." She eyed me with suspicion. Andrew sat next to me, watching silently.

"We needed information," I explained.

She blew out a column of smoke. My eyes followed it as it floated in the direction of a framed poster of a man. A banner read *Tony Stewart*. I turned my eyes back to her.

"You all could've come to me. But you didn't. You came *at* me," she declared. "You always want to make me out to be the bad guy, but I'm not the bad guy. You need to look at your own actions, your own behavior, like Dr. Phil says. Don't blame your parents for how your life turned out. My friend Ginger, here in the building, she's like my adopted daughter. She's nicer to me than you ever were. She respects what I teach her. She's a little older than you, but she's like a little child. I've taught her everything about this world! When she was young, she got put in an institution, where they didn't teach her anything! She didn't get the good public-school education you kids got! She's schizophrenic. Worse than you ever were—gets the voices and the whole nine yards. A hardcore mental! She'll tell you how kind I am—how I help all these drunks and mentals in this building. I'm the most generous person here. Don't come at me about the past! The past is the past! You can't blame me for your problems!"

"I don't want it to be like that, Mom. I just want information." I could feel pain in my jaw as I clamped my mouth shut. I knew I had to present my words in a way that would please her, regardless of the impact on me.

"Whadya ya need to know, hon? I told you who your dad is . . ." She trailed off. She ground out the stump of her cigarette in a red plastic ashtray and shook another from the pack.

"I need details, Mom. I want to try to find him."

We left with a full name and a short list of autobiographical details. It'd taken hours, but we'd extracted the information that I hoped would help me find my real dad.

# CHAPTER ELEVEN

WHERE ARE WE? Ah, 2013. A few more years had slipped by. You've gotta understand PMDD. It isn't impulsive. It's methodical.

I remember reading somewhere that most suicides combine a transitory mood with access to lethal means. Not PMDD. Andrew controlled my medication so I couldn't try to overdose. He'd locked up his guns. I'd stop eating and drinking for days to try to kill myself. I mean, not drinking water for three days straight isn't exactly impulsive. It's very freaking deliberate. Then my period would start, and I'd be like, "Wow, what was I thinking? I feel so much better now."

I'd learned when I'd been inpatient that Local Hospital had an intensive outpatient therapy program. I called and made an appointment.

"Hi, I'm Moonbeam, the therapist in charge of intake," said the wispy blonde on the day I arrived at the hospital. "I see you've been inpatient here. How wonderful that you're considering our outpatient program. Let's see. Oh, we don't have anything down for your level of education. How far did you go in school?"

"Um, I have a bachelor's degree," I said.

"What did you study?"

"Philosophy."

"Oh, I love Sartre! And Jung—brilliant. Existentialism. The Left Bank. Good stuff!" she cooed.

"Um, actually, I liked analytical philosophy more than the continental stuff. Logic was really my thing. I wrote one paper on Camus, but that was it—," I tried to explain. I'd never read Jung. Psychology was boring, indistinct, tedious.

"A paper on Camus? Awesome! I love *The Stranger*."

I tried to play along. "I thought *The Myth of Sisyphus* was pretty good."

"I haven't read that." She closed her mouth, and widened her eyes.

"Well, it's been awhile for me. I haven't read any philosophy books in years," I said.

"There you go! There's your problem!"

"Huh?"

"You've gotten away from your passion! You're a lost soul!" Moonbeam cried.

"Uh—"

"You need to pick up your books again. Dive in! That's why you're depressed!"

And she was off, pursuing a diatribe that sounded vaguely like disembodied consonants over the tinkling of wind chimes. It was awkward, but not strange. It had always been this way when talking to therapists.

I'd say I experienced *123* and the therapist or psychiatrist would respond that I had *actually* experienced *XYZ*, but because I was so depressed, or so anxious, or so anxious and depressed, that I couldn't see *XYZ*, and I mistook it for *123*. They spread their misinterpretations like an inverted map over my consciousness. They accused me of living in cities I'd never visited, like Selfsabotageville.

Moonbeam finally ran out of fuel. "We don't have an opening in our outpatient program right now," she said as she let her shoulders drop. "I can add your name to the waitlist."

I was halfway out the door by the time she said waitlist. As she spoke the word, my cadence turned to a run.

※

"I think I might have this premenstrual dysphoric disorder I read about," I cautiously offered my hypothesis to my psychiatrist, Dr. Boatbill, when I saw her.

"Your mood is still down?" she countered.

"Yes, I wanted to die until two days after my period started."

"We can increase your Effexor to the maximum dose."

"I think the Effexor is making me feel worse. Since I started taking it, my chest hurts and I feel dizzy."

"That's your anxiety. We can increase the Ativan while increasing the Effexor."

Often, Andrew came with me to my appointments. He was equally insistent that my depression correlated one to one with my menstrual cycle. Dr. Boatbill vacillated between either pretending we hadn't spoken or saying things like, "Well, even if you do have severe PMS, this is the protocol for PMS." And she'd offer another drug or two. She wouldn't speak the acronym PMDD.

"Anything else?" Dr. Boatbill would ask near the end of each appointment.

"Yes! Twilah won't pick up her phone during the day! I get so worried," Andrew would say.

Dr. Boatbill would turn her head in my direction. "Why won't you answer your phone?"

"I hate being interrupted. I can't multitask. It's confusing—"

Dr. Boatbill interrupted, "You need to answer the phone when Andrew calls. You have to understand that your illness causes him concern." She ended her rebuke with a stare, which made me divert my eyes to my lap.

"I know, but I'm not going to off myself at work." I shook my head. "I can't concentrate when my phone keeps ringing. I can't handle interruptions! I get paid to do my job, not talk on the phone to my husband. And we've been told we can't take personal calls at work."

"You have to understand that with your illness, you've given him reason to worry. At least respond to his texts." She continued to stare at me.

*Why does his need to bother me supersede my need to concentrate?* Concentration and focus were calming. *Why is it okay to upset my calm? Aren't they both supposed to be helping me stay calm?* But I kept my mouth closed. Clearly this wasn't up for discussion. And I was outnumbered.

She gave me Prozac, Celexa, Lexapro, Wellbutrin, Effexor, Cymbalta, and more. She dispensed benzos without hesitation. She augmented these treatments with antipsychotics and antiepileptics, on the premise that as "boosters" and mood stabilizers they'd address the cyclical nature of my depression.

The drugs she handed me always made me more sick and sad. I'd say as much to her, and she'd deny the possibility. "Your depression causes depression," she'd state. "You have a brain illness. You'll probably have to take medication for the rest of your life. You need to accept that."

⁂

*Boatbill didn't consider any kind of attention problem or sensory issue when you complained about your inability to multitask, or when you complained about how your concentration suffered when you were interrupted. I won't say I would've considered autism, but I certainly would have sent you to be evaluated for ADHD.*

Huh? Oh, you say that now. By this time, I had a mountain of medical records saying I was depressed, anxious, and a trauma victim. Victim, you hear me? Not survivor. Case closed. A mountain of records had been created by people who'd spent very little time interacting with me. By psychiatric or therapeutic standards, I was a typical hot mess of a woman ruined forever by trauma. Why investigate further?

You see how that works? I'd spent years trying to get a therapist or doctor to listen to me about my trauma, and they didn't want to hear it. But once they did hear it, they couldn't see past it. It defined me. I was nothing more than a reactive limbic system.

◈

I pushed the blade of the rotary cutter through the merlot-red cotton I'd arranged on the cutting table. I touched the tip of my index finger to each square I'd cut from the swath. The fabric was soft and smooth.

I moved the squares carefully over the gold and bronze background until they were aligned in perfect symmetry. I smiled, satisfied with my creation. I stepped away and opened the window. "Hi, Chuffies!" I sang to the squirrels who circled the base of the huge oak tree. *Chuff, chuff, chuff,* they replied.

I inhaled the peace I felt in the moment. *May this equanimity last.* I breathed the small prayer. It didn't.

I signed up for a different intensive outpatient group therapy program. I arrived a few minutes early and pushed my $500 down payment across the desk to the receptionist. "Have a seat in there." She pointed toward a small room decorated with posters.

I took a seat in a hard, plastic chair and inspected the walls around me. Big blue letters spelled out the word *Ecstasy* above a portrait of a woman. The woman's organs were exposed, and a sidebar detailed the effects of the drug on each of them. Lung failure, liver damage—my perusal was interrupted when an older white man entered the room.

"Hello, I'm Fred. I'm the therapist who leads this group. Here's a pen. Grab a form from the stack near the window and fill it out while we're waiting for everyone else to arrive."

I ignored the pen he offered and instead pulled one from my purse. I didn't like to touch strange objects.

*Name: Twilah*
*Positive statement about yourself: I'm a great dog mother*
*On a scale of 1-10, how depressed are you today: 8*
*How anxious: 7*

*List your medications: Cymbalta, Prozac, lorazepam, birth control*
*Are you taking them as prescribed? Yes*
*Psychiatrist name: Dr. Feather Boatbill*
*Do you have a therapist? No*
*Are you having thoughts of suicide? Yes*
*Can you promise the group to not carry out suicide? No*

Fifteen minutes after the scheduled start time, no one else had arrived. Fred and I spoke one on one. "I'm honestly glad nobody else showed up," I said. "I have a really hard time with groups. I can't explain it, really. I'm okay with people one on one, but groups are really overwhelming. They make me superanxious."

"Are you anxious at other times too?"

"Sometimes, but I'm always anxious in groups. My other problem is that I have something called PMDD. It means I get really depressed in the two weeks before my period."

"You can learn to control your anxiety," Fred said. "Start by listening to *blah-blah-blah*. It's a type of musical composition that affects the brainwaves associated with anxiety."

I couldn't follow all he'd said, but I pretended to understand so that he wouldn't get angry at me for asking him to repeat himself. Instead, I asked him to write down his suggestion. People didn't get as angry when I asked them to write things down. *Binaural beats*, I read on the scrap of paper he handed me. I liked that he'd offered a nonpharmaceutical recommendation.

That night, I downloaded a Binaural Beats MP3. I placed my earbuds in my ears and lay back onto my pillow. I felt my eyes darting from side to side in response to the pulsating tones, intended to facilitate relaxation. My stomach fluttered with what felt like the wingbeats of moths as my anxiety increased.

Two days later, I was back in Fred's domain. This time, five other patients arranged themselves in the chairs that lined the walls of the room.

I watched the shaggy head of a woman as it bobbed up and

down. She'd aim her bleary eyes at Fred, then seconds later her head would fall to her chest.

"Karen, are you doing okay?" Fred asked.

"Uhhhh," she replied.

"Karen, are you having a hard time staying awake?"

"Yaaaaa."

"Did you take medication? What did you take?" asked Fred.

"ZaaaNaaaaax," she slurred.

"How much Xanax?

"Ayyyyyyy."

"Eight?" asked Fred.

"Yaaaaa."

I'd worked fatality claims when I'd been in insurance. Each contact with a surviving spouse or family member had left me near tears. Minutes before, I'd watched Karen park next to me and stumble into the building. I waited to see if Fred would say anything to her about driving. The session concluded without Fred saying a word. I watched her vehicle swerve away.

I knew I should've spoken up. A dense cloud of condemnation encircled my thoughts. *You are bad for not opening your mouth and objecting to her intoxicated driving. You are bad because you didn't stand up for what's right. You are bad because you let your anxiety keep you from speaking.*

By the third session, I realized I was one of only two people attending the group who didn't have a substance abuse problem.

"Yeah, I'd been clean for three days. I was doin' pretty good. But then my oldest girl's daddy, Keith, came over, and he had some crystal, so I bought it offa 'im. But then my littlest baby didn't have diapers, and I didn't have no more money. So, I left the house to do a trick, and my neighbor called the law cuz she heard my baby—" A woman with greasy blond hair was telling the tale. I felt my hands balling into fists. My fingernails dug into my palms.

"I'm really having a hard time being sympathetic to these people's immoral choices." I'd cut her off.

"Drug addiction isn't an immoral choice. It's a disease," Fred rushed to correct me. "It's like any other disease. You need to understand that."

As soon as I saw his mouth close, I jumped in again. "It's *not* like any other disease. You don't know you have an addiction *disease* until you take a drug that you know damn well is addictive. That's *not* like other disease processes. You deliberately do something you've been told not to do, and only then do you have symptoms. I do have sympathy for people who become addicts because they've had drugs forced on them—like people enslaved by traffickers or psychiatric patients. But you're asking me to feel sympathy for someone when their choice results in a defenseless minor child being left unattended? I don't motherfucking think so. They're like fucking pedophiles, putting their pleasure seeking before the needs of their children for safety."

Fred's eyes narrowed, and his voice rose. "You're wrong. Stop being judgmental, and start being supportive. Addiction is a disease!"

Weeks passed. I became more and more angry and more and more sad. Chastened by Fred, I kept my mouth closed even when the most terrible tales were told by the addicts. But that wasn't enough. Fred lectured me at each meeting on how I needed to empathize with the struggles of these people whose motivations and behaviors I could not understand.

I broke through the wall of sound and spoke again. "I think this Prozac's making me angrier. I've taken it before, and every single time it's made me feel angry."

"It's your depression that's making you angry, not your medication," he replied.

"No, I really think it's the Prozac. This has happened every single time I've taken it. I don't like it."

"You're not the first person to feel angry," Fred retorted.

"I know," I responded after a pause. I hadn't said I was the first person to feel angry. Why had he said that? I reconfigured my words. "I don't like it. I don't want to take Prozac anymore. It's interfering with my spiritual goals. I'm Buddhist. And in Buddhism, while anger is okay under certain circumstances, expressing anger this way is regarded as unskilled."

"First of all, anger is a symptom of depression. That's why you're angry," he paused. "Listen to me. Your anger is *not* because of your medication. It's because of your depression. And anger is a natural emotion. You need to accept it. Your problem is that you suppress your feelings. You're too analytical. You overthink things—that's your response to trauma. You need to *feel* more, be more *expressive*. Accepting your anger is the first step."

I opened my mouth to speak, but I wasn't fast enough. I'd been analytical long before I'd been traumatized.

"I've been treating trauma for over thirty years. I'm somewhat of an *expert* in my field," he puffed the word *expert* with the force of a boxer's punch.

From my car, I left a tear-choked voicemail for the program director. "Hi, um, this is Twilah Hiari, and I'm in the outpatient program. I'm not going to be attending the group anymore. I can't sit and listen to the things the addicts say. I can't handle it. So, yeah, I won't be coming back. Thank you. Bye."

When I checked my voicemail two days later, there was a message asking me to come in and pay the balance of my bill.

⁓⦆

*Fred wouldn't consider the possibility that your anger could be due to a known side effect of Prozac. I'm a little disappointed by that.*

No, he wouldn't. Again, it's like these people, *you* people, become completely illiterate when it comes to reading FDA warning labels or even a WebMD page. Ego can be a real bitch that way.

# CHAPTER TWELVE

*May all beings be endowed with happiness. May all beings be free from suffering. May all beings never be separated from happiness. May all beings abide in equanimity, undisturbed by the eight worldly concerns.* – Four Immeasurables, Buddhist prayer

I LOWERED MY eyelids until I could only see a sliver of flickering light from the candle on the altar. I felt a small point of pressure in my back and knew it was the paw of my Golden Pyrenees as she stretched out on her cushion behind me. The breath flowed into my abdomen as my lips pulled into a smile. She was my constant companion in meditation.

Days later, any semblance of peace was gone. My brain felt like it was splitting open. I was titrating off the Cymbalta, and the withdrawal was insane. I'd get so dizzy while sitting at my desk working that I'd slide off the chair and onto the floor. I'd been taking Cymbalta and Prozac, but I was trying to get off the Cymbalta and onto Prozac alone.

*That seems like an odd change. From a newer SNRI to an older SSRI.*

Huh? Yeah, it was. The reason for the change is because I'd started wanting to have a baby. Dr. Boatbill had told me that Prozac was a safer drug than Cymbalta for pregnancy.

***But you mentioned before that one of the reasons you'd gotten together with Andrew is because he didn't want kids.***

Yeah, that's how I knew I had gone completely off the deep end hormone-wise. I wanted a kid, which is completely irrational.

***I think wanting a baby is a normal desire.***

No, it's not freaking normal. Not for *me.* I've always hated kids, especially screaming babies. But I'd just started having these feelings. I'd see visions of myself with this big pregnant belly, and I'd get this sensation of craving. I can't describe it. It was just a longing, a desire. I knew rationally that there's zero appeal in changing diapers, listening to constant wailing, or getting puked on. But those thoughts didn't change these images that kept appearing in my mind. I'd never experienced an impulse so strong and irrational, except for the suicidal impulses. It's crazy how powerful it was.

But really, you can't make the case that wanting to procreate is rational. Not successfully, you can't. The only thing you can appeal to is the continuation of the human species, and at seven billion plus, we're not exactly facing a shortage.

Explain how it's rational to create a human being you've never met, who arrives with any personality or condition, ability or disability. You know absolutely nothing about them in advance, other than that they'll share some of your genes. Based on this alone, you agree to support them for eighteen years, minimum. *Minimum,* you hear me? Because if things don't go as you hope, you might have to support them for a lot longer.

And it'll cost you a lot of money. I read somewhere that it costs an average of a quarter of a million dollars, which you probably don't have sitting around in the bank. Your kid might turn out to be an accountant, or they might turn out to be a serial killer. They might end up a minister or a child molester. Or a child-molesting minister. They might end up curing cancer. Or they might end up chronically suicidal until the day they finally blow their brains out in front of you. And there's very little you can do about any of that, despite how much you tell yourself otherwise. You have to be willing to accept any of those possibilities and infinitely more. I don't know how many people can honestly say they're ready for that.

So please, tell me how that's a rational decision. No, actually—don't even try. Because you can't, and I don't want to get distracted and confused while you blabber on. So, back to my original point. Those are some of the circumstances underlying what happened next—Cymbalta withdrawal and a crazy hormone surge.

---

"I need help please. I don't want to die." I spoke the words through a mesh screen in a glass window.

The woman behind the glass waved at the chairs behind me. "Ambulances take priority over walk-ins," she said. I watched her lips closely to better grasp her words. "There're two ambulances on the way. Once they're checked in, you'll be next."

I sat in a chair and sobbed. A television hung in the corner, filling the room with noise. I put in my earbuds and sat staring at the wall of lockers in front of me. An hour passed. No ambulances came.

I got up and whispered through the mesh, "Will I get checked in soon? I need help."

"I told you there are ambulances coming, and they get checked in first." The young woman's voice was loud. She seemed angry.

"So, what if I run into the street and get hit by a car? Can I get checked in then?"

"That's up to you," she said with a shrug. She swiveled her chair and offered her back to me.

Two and a half hours later, another woman came out. She asked me to follow her to a room. I curled up on a bed, buried my head under a blanket, and fell asleep.

For a day and a half, I sat in tearful meditation. I had a roommate with whom I didn't interact. Meals and medications were brought to us, but the staff who brought them didn't say anything to me. On the third day, a large black man with a Nigerian accent woke me in the middle of the night. I put on my glasses and squinted at his blue scrubs as he leaned over me. "They're moving you to another room," he said. "Follow me."

I followed him down a long hallway to another room, where I could see the outline of a woman sleeping on one of two narrow beds. I lay down on the vacant bed and slept.

Late the next morning, a pink-skinned woman with glasses that looked like they were pinching her nose stormed into my room.

"You need to start following the rules around here," she said.

"Huh?"

"You didn't go to morning group, and you didn't go to breakfast. You have to follow the rules!"

"Nobody told me about any of that," I responded.

"Well, now you know!" she shot back. She turned and walked out into the hallway.

I stayed in my room and cried. I didn't want to go out and be yelled at by more staff. I just wanted to die. Throughout the day, techs peeked their heads in the door, made notes on their clipboards, and left. I watched other patients pass by as they paced the hallways. No one spoke to me except for twice a day when a tech would tell me to go to the nurses' station and get my meds.

By evening, I'd become hungry. I crept down the hall and saw a whiteboard covered in writing. I scanned down until I saw *Dinner 6:00 p.m.* printed in black dry-erase Magic Marker.

At five fifty-five, I left my room. I queued up at the end of a line of patients that had formed in the hallway. I stepped farther and farther back from the people in front of me. They were talking too loudly and moving around too much. Their voices hurt my head, and I didn't want their agitated movements to propel their bodies into me. Two metal double doors opened with a pneumatic squeal that made me wince.

The patients marched down a hall to the cafeteria. I kept my eyes on the woman in front of me so I could figure out how the process worked. I'd always been intimidated by cafeterias. At the high schools I'd attended, the big rooms had been so off-putting that I'd usually refused to enter them at all. I knew that wasn't an option here. I'd already been yelled at for not following the rules. I focused my attention on the woman in front of me and mimicked everything she did. My stomach lurched at the thought of making a mistake or having to ask a question. I took my tray and looked for a seat as far away from everyone else as possible.

A few seats away, three loud, obese white women kept looking in my direction and muttering. I could hear bits and pieces of their rant. The word "bitch" was repeated with enthusiasm. I realized they were talking about me and looked away. They became bored by their intimidation game and turned their conversation to the relative merits of meth versus bath salts as weight-loss aids.

My period started the next morning. I crept to the nurses' station to ask for a pad. Several nurses sat staring at computer screens. I stood directly in front of a nurse with my hands clasped at my pelvis and eyes pointed down at the counter. The nurse didn't look up.

"Excuse me," I said quietly to a brown-skinned nurse with thick, braided hair.

Her eyes stayed fixed on her screen.

"Excuse me," I tried again.

"We're at shift change. You're going to have to wait," she snapped. Her accent sounded vaguely Caribbean.

I went back to my room and cried some more. I used the rough towels I'd found in the bathroom to clean up the blood that was now all over my pants.

Anger churned in my stomach. It rose up my chest, then into my throat. My skin stung as my sock-clad feet hammered against the cold white tile and propelled me up the hallway. I stood in front of the nurses' station again. The nurses continued talking amongst themselves. Their voices sounded like the gaggles of geese that congregated in the park near my home during the summer—squawk-squawking that made no sense.

"Hello!" I yelled. "Am I invisible, or are you unprofessional?"

A big nurse with pressed hair looked up. Her mouth hung open as she regarded me. "Well, well—," she stammered.

"I need a fucking pad. And am I ever going to see a doctor? Or anyone? I want treatment now, or I want to go home!"

"Oh, oh, I'm so sorry," she replied. "Let me get you some pads."

She unlocked a closet and dug some out.

"You haven't seen anyone because you haven't gone to groups," she said. "Let me see who your social worker is—oh, I'll have Angela come get you."

"Who the fuck is Angela, and where is she going to get me from?"

"Angela's your social worker. You can go to the group room, and she'll come get you," she said as she pointed to a room across the hall.

I became angrier when I entered the room and heard the television blaring from the corner. Then I became angry at myself for being so angry.

The three fat pasty-faced women from the cafeteria sat around a table. They glared at me as they hovered protectively over a Winnie the Pooh outline in a coloring book. I sat in a corner and stared back hard.

"The fuck you want?" I growled.

They dropped their bloodshot eyes.

"Tah-uh."

I glanced up at the sound I could barely hear over the television.

A frail looking young white woman was standing in the doorway.

"Huh, did you say Twilah?" I asked.

"Yes."

I walked toward her. Outside of the room, I could hear.

"Hi, I'm Angela. Let's step into this room." I followed her hand as it pointed to a tiny room with a sofa and a chair. She waved for me to sit down on the sofa.

"What brings you here?" she asked.

"Every goddamned month I want to die. I'm sick of it. Every goddamned month I get so that I can't do anything. I get up and shower, and I try to do things, but I can't. I start crying, and then I go back to bed. I hate it."

"Well, you're depressed. And despite your depression, sometimes you just have to get up and do things anyway. No more excuses! You have to do what you have to do. And sooner or later, you're going to have to get help for your PTSD. I saw your records from the outpatient group. You need to deal with that. It's not going to go away on its own," she lectured as she shot a stare at me. I looked down and began to cry. I cried for several minutes before Angela told me I could go to my room.

A few minutes later, a tech retrieved me and led me to another room. "Wait here, and your doctor will be in shortly," she said before turning to leave. I began counting the colors of the book bindings on the shelf across from me. Seven red, nineteen brown, four green—

A minute into my count, a man in a plaid shirt entered the room. He smiled and introduced himself as Dr. Pleasant. I spent thirty minutes telling Dr. Pleasant about my PMDD and ever-increasing anxiety. He seemed to listen. He wasn't mean or scary. He didn't talk too loudly or too softly.

"Have you tried mirtazapine?" he asked.

I struggled to spell the word in my head. It didn't sound familiar. "Uh, no, I don't think so."

"Well, then let's try that with some clonazepam for your anxiety."

"I don't like the way benzos make me feel. I can't put my finger on it, but I think they make me feel sicker and sadder," I tried to explain.

"You'll still need some way to deal with your anxiety. Let's do a very low dose. Let's try a quarter of a milligram twice a day." He looked at me for approval. His voice was soft. I decided I could trust him.

"Okay. I'll try it."

By afternoon, I'd begun to feel a little better. I went to the nurses' station and asked if I could see Angela again. A few minutes later, Angela led me back to the room where we'd first spoken.

"I want to talk to you about what you said earlier. It's really bothering me. I know that I need to do what I'm supposed to do. I want very badly to do what I'm supposed to do. I'd like to work. I'd like to keep my house clean. I'd like to walk my dogs. I'd like to cook dinner. But I can't, despite how much I want to. And I've been trying for over a decade to get help for my PTSD. I keep getting dismissed or shut down in therapy. That's how I ended up here. I'm desperate."

I took a breath and tried to form more words in my head.

"Your remark that I just had to get up and do things despite the PMDD was the worst thing you could've said," I continued. "If I could do the things I need to do, I wouldn't be here getting charged two grand a day to be ignored by staff and bullied by the women of the trailer park mafia."

"Well, you're going to have to assert yourself," Angela said.

"Jesus Christ! That's what I'm doing now. It's what I've been trying to learn how to do for years! I can't figure it out on my own. I want help! I'm not lazy. I'm sick. And I'm sick of being sick. But you know what? I feel better now, and I want to go home. Can I just go home?"

Three hours later, I was discharged from the hospital.

***

*Did you have any friends in your life at this time?*

No. I still hadn't made any friends since college. I had no idea how to make friends outside of classrooms.

*What about family? Were you still talking to your brothers?*

I hadn't talked to Glen since we'd confronted our mom. He'd disappeared. I talked to Jeffrey occasionally. He'd update me on his new girlfriend or new wife or new divorce or new childbirth or new work situations. He rarely asked about my life. He always said I was a great listener. Everyone I met said I was a great listener. And I was. And I was glad to be. But I guess no one considered that I only listened, smiled, nodded, and agreed because I had no idea how to insert or assert myself in a conversation—that I had no idea how to ask for what I needed.

# CHAPTER THIRTEEN

I PULLED THE cotton fabric from the dryer. The heat radiating from the cloth warmed my fingers, which, like my toes, were always ice cold. I carefully folded each piece before taking the stack upstairs.

I rested the iron on each piece and listened to the soft sizzle that arose as the last bits of moisture were released into the air. I closed my eyes and tried to recall one of the many patterns that had filled my dreams the night before. I butted a cedar-colored quarter against its raspberry shaded counterpart. I admired the pair as the hues seemed to radiate from the table. The colors now imbued the pattern that had formed in my mind. I rested in the hues and the tranquility they brought.

Two weeks later, I could no longer pull myself from bed. I called Local Hospital and said I wanted to try electroconvulsive therapy. Dr. Pintalabios had pushed ECT the second time I'd been under her care, but I'd refused. Huh? Yeah, I'd been inpatient at Local Hospital more times than I have time to tell. As soon as I'd refused, she'd discharged me. Later, when I'd seen the bills for each session of

ECT, Dr. Pintalabios' motivation became clearer. Each session cost hundreds of dollars, and a good portion of that charge went to the doctor. I'd been afraid of ECT when Dr. Pintalabios had tried to sell it to me. I'd read it could cause memory loss and brain damage.

But with the PMDD raging, my judgment was distorted. And I thought there might be some memories I wouldn't mind losing.

Becky, the nurse who coordinated the ECT treatments, told me that I needed to agree to another inpatient stay if I wanted to get treatment started right away. I signed the commitment sheet.

This time my doctor was a Dr. Iyilik. He spoke softly in an accent I'd never heard before, so I had to stare extra hard at his mouth to understand him.

"Why are you here today? I see that you've been here before," he said.

"I can't handle being sick anymore. My husband's about to lose his job because he misses so much work over me being sick. Between my medical bills and my lost income, we had to file for bankruptcy last year. I *have* to get well."

Dr. Iyilik nodded. "Most patients' moods improve a lot with ECT. I think it will help you get better." His soft voice was calming.

My first treatment was scheduled for five a.m. I got up at four, did my prostrations, said my dedications, and sat for twenty minutes in meditation. I counted off more prayers as I waited for the mental health tech to take me downstairs.

I stared across the giant room. It was filled with beds that rested on locked wheels. Thin curtains were drawn closed between the beds as IVs were inserted into the hands or arms of the other patients.

"Hi, I'm Clara!" chirped the red-haired nurse. "Where do you want your IV?" she asked as she grabbed my hand.

"No, no, not there." My stomach jumped as the words poured forth. "Not my hand. That freaks me out."

She dropped my hand. "Oh, it's easier that way, but I can do your arm if you want."

I pointed at a spot in my inner elbow, and Clara jabbed at me with the needle. "You're a hard stick!" she declared before withdrawing the tip. Andrew had always told me I was an easy stick. I watched the blood begin to pool under my skin. By the fourth jab, I'd begun to cry. She'd been chattering nonstop as she aimed the instrument at my vein.

"Am I hurting you?"

"Yes!" I yelled before lapsing back into silence. The pain and her incessant speech were driving my mind away from the world around me and into the refuge of my thoughts. I gripped a printed image of the Medicine Buddha on my stomach and closed my eyes.

A mask was placed over my nose and mouth. I inhaled a strange scent as I drifted off.

"Toe ah, Toe ah," chanted Chatty Clara.

*Is she saying my name?* I opened my eyes.

"Whew, that was a big one! Your Buddha went flying! I had to pick him up off the floor!" She cackled.

"Okaaay," I murmured. My face was soaked in tears, but I felt entirely free of all emotions.

I woke up later that afternoon. I'd slept for several hours but still felt exhausted. I went to a lounge and called Andrew.

"How'd the treatment go?" he asked.

"Huh?"

"How did the ECT go?"

"Uh, I don't know. Okay, I guess. I'm so tired."

"That's probably just the anesthesia."

"What?"

"It's probably the anesthesia," Andrew repeated.

"Yeah, that's what they told me."

I went to the groups, hopeful that I'd finally learn the coping skills I'd been wanting to learn for decades. In each group, I sat silently, fighting to extract meaning from the words that swirled around me. In the art group, the therapist asked each of us to explain the meanings behind our drawings.

A woman spoke. "Mine's about how I'm a bad mom. I spend more money on pills than my kids."

"Oh, you're a good mom! You do your best. Don't beat yourself up. Your kids love you," the other patients cheered. I picked out the phrases before the sounds of the many speakers started to flow together in a river of clotted consonants. Rage curdled in my chest and pushed at the bottom of my throat. I pressed my teeth into my lower lip and left the room.

When I woke up the next morning, my thoughts turned to the addicts on the ward. Hunger gnawed at me, but I didn't want to leave my room to get my food tray. I might see the loudest addict from last night's group. I could see her stringy brown hair hanging around her face as she warbled on about smoking this and snorting that. I visualized my fist arching into her throat.

I stalked out of my room and began pacing in rapid laps around the ward. I could feel small jolts of pain in my shins as my feet slapped the floor. I fingered an invisible mala, or Buddhist prayer beads, and counted the glowing red exit sign each time I passed. I'd reached fifty-three laps when I heard the locked door of the ward click open.

"Oh, I see you are exercising this morning!" Dr. Iyilik exclaimed as he crossed the threshold.

"Huh?" I bought time to process his words.

"How are you doing this morning?"

"Can I go get some notes from my room?" I had ignored his question. I had to stay focused.

"Sure," he answered.

I returned with my notes, and Dr. Iyilik signaled us into an unoccupied room.

"I want to go home," I read from my notes. "I cannot heal in the presence of these drug abusers. It's taking all of my energy to not give them a piece of my mind. Energy I don't have. It makes no sense that I should have to go to groups with them. Would you put a rape survivor in a group made up of rapists? I don't feel safe."

Dr. Iyilik nodded. "I wouldn't have chosen to combine the addiction recovery group with the mental health group. That decision was made by someone else—someone in administration. You should write to the administrators about it when you get home.

Are you feeling better otherwise?"

"Yeah," I lied.

"Then I'll approve your discharge," he said.

When I arrived home, I went straight to the bathroom. "I'm having terrible diarrhea," I said to Andrew.

"Uh-oh," he said. "That's bad news with all the antibiotics you've been taking."

A few weeks earlier, a physician assistant who worked with Dr. Vite had prescribed some antibiotics to treat an episode of bronchitis. Two weeks after that, I'd taken another round of antibiotics to treat an abscess that had appeared on my skin.

After I told Andrew about the diarrhea, he drove me to his lab and handed me a plastic receptacle. After the fecal contents were transferred to a cup and analyzed, I learned I had a Clostridium difficile (C. diff) infection.

"C. diff is a serious infection," Andrew explained. "It can be fatal. The first-line treatment is usually Flagyl. I don't know what they're going to give you since you can't tolerate Flagyl."

The last time I'd taken Flagyl, my eyes had lost the ability to focus and measure distance. The optical problems had left me dizzy and disoriented.

"The second-line treatment is vancomycin," Denise, the physician assistant explained. "We'll skip to that since you had a reaction to Flagyl."

"Okay then." I nodded.

*You were stomping around the ward in a rage state, and Dr. Iyilik thought you were exercising?*

Ha-ha, yeah. I was like two inches from a full-on meltdown. But you reminded me. You want to know what else Dr. Iyilik was wrong about? I was on lamotrigine at the time. Dr. Boatbill had added it in because even though she didn't believe in PMDD, she'd finally acknowledged that my depression was cyclical—precisely cyclical. She'd been witnessing it for years. She prescribed lamotrigine off label as a mood stabilizer. Her thought process was that it would balance my moods over the course of the month.

Well, the lamotrigine didn't do shit for my mood, but it caused really bad pain in both my Achilles tendons. The pain started within days of me taking the drug, and nothing else in my life had changed. I told Dr. Iyilik about my pain and my suspicion that the lamotrigine had caused it. He called a hospital pharmacist upstairs to talk to me.

"I looked up the probability that lamotrigine is causing your tendon pain. That's a side effect that only affects 1 percent of people, so that's not the reason for your pain," the pharmacist declared.

I didn't say anything when she spoke because I was too busy wondering what that translated to. How many people took lamotrigine? If her estimate of tendon pain affecting 1 percent of patients was correct, and one million people took lamotrigine, then up to ten thousand people would have tendon pain as a side effect. That's a lot of people!

But doctors and pharmacists, they don't think like that. They have a real hard time with perspective. I call it being blinded by improbability. They conflate *statistically improbable* with *impossible event that I'm never gonna see*. And that's a big problem for a small number of real people.

It so happens that I'd had the same tendon pain when I'd taken Zocor, a cholesterol drug Dr. Vite had prescribed, so this wasn't the first time this had happened. After I stopped the lamotrigine—against Dr. Boatbill's orders—the tendon pain went away. So, you figure that one out. But you know what my medical record says about it? It says: *Patient complains of tendon pain, probably from excessive walking.*

Because doing a quarter mile in laps around the psych ward is excessive walking when I used to run 10K races.

*There's a lot of tension of an us versus them variety. Us being you, and them being drug users. But you were on drugs, don't you see that?*

Huh? Of course I do. Listen. I hated the PMDD mood swings, but I was willing to do anything not to die. The difference is first, I'd been trying to dump psych drugs for years, but the authorities, the doctors that is, kept lying and telling me they were good for me.

Nobody's telling addicts that meth or heroin or whatever is good for them. Nobody. And another difference is that drug addicts hurt other people. Always. The idea that drug abuse is a victimless crime is one of the biggest lies ever told. A person who crosses the line of serious drug abuse can't be trusted, not until they're completely clean. I was scared to be on the ward with them. I felt extra vigilant. Because around addicts, you always have to be ready to fight, to defend yourself because they're all about taking. They'll destroy anything that stands between them and whatever they want to take.

Another thing that's messed up is that these addicts were getting preferential treatment. Because if you do drugs, then people assume you've had a shitty life and you get all this sympathy. Like "Boohoo, what drove you to this?" I'd done so well in terms of education and conformity to middle-class expectations that people refused to believe I'd ever lived through adversity.

But don't you see how psychiatrists are the worst drug dealers on the planet? They're more intimidating than the gangbangers I'd run into back home. The dealers back in the 'hood, when they'd offered me drugs, I'd said, "Naw, I ain't about that shit." And they left me alone. Not the dealers in the medical offices. They didn't take no for an answer. Like fucking rapists.

*I can't say I disagree with your assessment. Let's talk about the ECT. Your first session was intense.*

Yeah, I think their settings were off or something. I don't think my seizure was supposed to be that big. But I figured if something had gone wrong, they would've told me. There I go assuming integrity—projecting my values onto other people.

I think that's when my brain injury started. And that's really a big deal. In Kansas, the statute of limitations for tort claims, like for bodily injury or medical malpractice, is two years. My first ECT treatment was on April 23, 2014, at five ten a.m. So, the clock was running. Tick-tock.

# CHAPTER FOURTEEN

THE FUR BENEATH my fingers was short and course. "Hey, honey, come meet me at The Rescue Center," I spoke into my phone.

"Are you serious?"

"Yeah, I'm serious. You gotta see this guy."

"Alright, I'm on my way," Andrew replied.

A few minutes later, Andrew walked into the back room of the shelter. "You want that?" he asked. He stared at the emaciated Chihuahua that stood cowering and quaking in my lap.

"Yes, I want him! He can wear shirts, and I can carry him around!"

"A small dog—really? A yippy-yappy dog?" Andrew sighed.

"If we train him right, he won't be yippy. I want him!"

"Okay," Andrew said with a slight shake of his head.

My hormones had exploded. Even after I'd bought him a drawer full of sweaters, the Chihuahua was not enough. My hormones were telling me I needed to have a human baby.

Andrew and I made an appointment with a doctor who specialized in reproductive endocrinology. See, Andrew had gotten fixed before we'd gotten married, so I knew we'd need medical intervention to achieve my newfound goal. That's how I met Dr. Fahrig.

I went to Dr. Fahrig with a plan of procreation in mind, but within a couple of visits, we changed course.

"Has your psychiatrist acknowledged that your depression is associated with your menstrual cycle?" she asked.

"Not really. She's seen that it is, but she won't call it PMDD."

"Well, I'll call it PMDD," Dr. Fahrig said. "Until we're ready for the IVF treatment, I think you should try going back on oral birth control. That helps some women with PMDD symptoms. If that doesn't work, we can consider other options."

I was now seeing Dr. Fahrig for PMDD and Dr. Iyilik for my psych drugs and ECT. I figured I'd try one last time to find a therapist, and I'd be set. I'd have a full team to help me get well.

The therapist's office was located inside a house about a mile away from mine. I entered through the back door. A mudroom opened into a kitchen. I picked up a clipboard that held the paperwork I'd been told would be waiting for me. Tea and mugs were set out on a small side table. I loved herbal tea, but I strode quickly past the mugs and into the adjacent room. I had to silence the noise first.

A discordant series of notes blasted from the speakers of a radio that rested on a shelf. I rotated the volume knob to zero. I hated NPR, especially *All Things Considered*. The sound effects sprinkled throughout the stories made me seethe. From that point forward, the first thing I did when I arrived for therapy was turn off the radio.

The sound of footsteps filled the room, and a tall, thin dark-haired woman peeked in. She looked ten or fifteen years older than me.

"Hi, are you Twilah?" she asked.

"Yes," I said as I stood up from a chair.

"I'm Grace. Come on up." I headed in the direction of her waving hand. We climbed wooden stairs and entered another small room. She waved at two chairs that sat side by side. I sat in the one nearest the window, taking care not to brush my skin against the rough fabric of the chair.

"What brings you here?" she asked as she positioned herself across from me.

"Um, a few years ago, I was a motivated and high-energy person. I had goals, and I worked to meet them. I was driven, and I was happy. I had a good job, and I was in really good shape. Now I fight to stay alive every month. I've been diagnosed with PMDD, which is premenstrual dysphoric disorder. I tried to tell therapists for years that my depression only comes with my period, but no one believed me. I'm getting treatment for that from a reproductive endocrinologist. Anyway, I've been told I have PTSD too, and that's what I hope you can help me with."

"It's good that you want to address those things. I think I'll be able to help you," Grace said with a small, slow nod. "But being driven isn't really a good thing. Driven people burn out. What's your educational background?"

"I have a bachelor's degree in philosophy from KU."

"That's practical!" she blurted with a laugh.

I felt tears rise up. I took a breath and tamped them down.

"Actually, it is," I countered. "It provides a great foundation for a legal education. I planned to go to law school afterward, even though my professors pushed me toward a PhD instead. I applied to seven law schools and got accepted to all of them. But I couldn't afford to go, even with the scholarships they offered. In terms of practicality, I've had good jobs in insurance, and my course of study never put me at a disadvantage there."

I paused, awed by the fact that I'd successfully stood up for myself. My words had come out exactly as I'd intended. I watched Grace raise her eyebrows.

The defense I'd offered had been true but incomplete. My professors *had* encouraged me to get a PhD in philosophy. But I knew I could never teach. I became confused when people lobbed questions at me. I couldn't think through complex questions and give complex answers, not when they were spoken. If the questions were written, and I could respond in writing, I could communicate perfectly well. That was the real reason I hadn't pursued a PhD, but I was too ashamed to admit to what I thought of as my secret stupidity.

Everything I'd said had been true. Despite generous scholarship offers, law school would've been hard to afford. But the foundational reason I hadn't gone hadn't been financial. I'd sat in on a class when I visited the University of Minnesota after I'd been accepted there. I'd immediately realized that the oral question and answer format of law school would be just as impossible to navigate as teaching.

"Tell me what you remember about your life starting from as young as you can recall. Who was in your life? What were things like?"

My mouth opened and closed with surprise. No one had ever asked me that before. I tipped my head back and recalled an image. There was a basement. The floor was shiny and grey. It felt cold and hard under my hands and knees. I watched small furry animals run in and out of transparent tubes and boxes. Hamsters? I described the images to Grace.

"How old were you in that house?" she asked.

I closed my eyes again. The house was what my mother had always called "the house on 60th." We'd lived there before Jeffrey was born, and he was about three and a half years younger than me. After the house on 60th, we'd moved to another house on a street called Tauromee. We'd lived there for a year. Jeffrey hadn't been born until we'd moved to a third house on a street called Hauser.

"Um, I must have been two and a half or younger," I deduced.

Grace's eyebrows rose again. "What other memories do you have?"

"That's all for that house. From the next house I have this memory that I really don't understand." I paused to focus on the rise and fall of my stomach. "I was in the bathroom, sitting on the counter by the sink. My older brother, Glen, was in the bathroom too. He told me to look in the mirror and say, 'Bloody Mary, Bloody Mary, Bloody Mary.' " I smashed my eyelids closed and replayed the scene.

"I remember a razor blade. I remember bright-red blood seeping under the closed bathroom door. The door was white. The floor was light beige with a triangle print. I remember my mom screaming. That's it. That's all." I turned my palms up and shrugged.

"Did you ever learn if that was a real event? Sometimes our minds create memories that aren't really memories."

"No. I asked my mom and Glen about it, but they both say nothing like that ever happened. What they do say is that Glen superglued my T-shirt to my skin and that I'd had to go to the hospital to get it unstuck."

"Glen sounds—I don't know—how did you think of yourself when you were young?"

"I wanted to be a boy when I was little. I remember thinking that as soon as I could work, I'd save up money to buy a sex change."

"You know why that is, right?"

I didn't know, so I shook my head and waited for her to tell me.

"It's because you grew up in a very sexist society."

I thought she was wrong. My desire to be a boy had lived apart from any sexism I had perceived around me. But I didn't speak. She'd stated her position clearly, and that signaled she'd be ready for a rapid verbal argument. And it no longer mattered. I'd grown out of wanting to be a boy.

&

*Even though you were still ashamed to admit the real reason you hadn't pursued more education, you'd gotten to a point where you could talk about your family. It's like your shame about them was gone. How'd you get to that point?*

Wait, wait, wait. I'd been trying to talk about my family for years, but nobody wanted to hear it. The difference is I could finally talk about them calmly. Meditation and dharma teachings, the teachings of the Buddha—that's what got me to that point. You see, many of the teachings emphasize how all humans are trying to be happy. But some humans make mistakes and do things that they think will make them happy, but those things actually cause more suffering. I'd forced myself to pay closer attention to other people, because I don't take anything on faith.

When I'd started looking hard at people's behaviors, I'd found that the teaching was true. People do crazy, irrational things, like drugs and human breeding, and then they're shocked when those things make them less happy in the long run or even in the short term. But I also saw that what I'd been doing before was looking at the *results* of people's actions, while completely overlooking their *motivations.*

Most people have a kind of blind spot when it comes to seeing that $X$ will lead to $Y$. And that's all I'd been able to see about people in the past—that they had a terrible problem identifying causal relationships. I'd thought, *All the people around me are insane* based on the horrible decisions I'd watched people make.

But cause and effect aren't clear to most people. They get blinded by emotions and pleasure seeking. So, back to my point—when I'd paid close attention, I'd seen that fundamentally, the teaching was true. We're all trying to be happy, but other people are more prone to making certain mistakes in attaining happiness because they can't fathom causal relationships or consequences and repercussions. Or they reject causal realities they *can* see because they magically override them with feelings. But even if they're blind regarding causation, or in total denial because of emotions, they're still trying to do the exact same thing I'm trying to do—be happy.

When I meditated on that for a long time, and internalized that teaching, I finally felt like I belonged in the world. And the shame evaporated. The shame had been about me having bad experiences that were so different from the experiences of anyone else I knew. It'd been about this tension between being the good person I knew I was and having had all this bad shit happen to me. It didn't make any sense, and I knew that irrational people, which is most people, would conflate the bad events outside of my control with some kind of inherent badness inside me.

I figured out this was a miscalculation people made to facilitate their own happiness. They couldn't look the world in the eye and acknowledge how unfair it is. It was too hard for them. And I understood. I'd felt the pain that comes from recognizing the world isn't just or fair. So, I started to forgive people for being so irrational and judging me because of their irrationality.

Having had that realization, I should've walked out of Grace's office and meditated even more. I mean, I should've meditated for years. I should've spent some serious time contemplating. But I didn't. Instead, I allowed this Western notion of therapy as the optimal path for mental change to supplant the value of the meditation practice that had already started to heal me and transform my mind.

But you know what's interesting? It turns out things would get so complicated that even the most rational person couldn't have anticipated the consequences.

# CHAPTER FIFTEEN

I WAS GETTING sicker. The C. diff had come back and the physician assistant Kelly, who was now my primary care provider, referred me to a gastroenterologist. The PA at the gastroenterology office, a woman named Soa, had instructed me to take another round of vancomycin for the infection.

One of my toenails had fallen off from a fungal infection. I told Kelly about it, and she started typing. After a minute, she said, "We usually prescribe terbinafine for toenail fungus, but that's contraindicated with amitriptyline. It could cause the amitriptyline to build up in your system and become more potent. But you're on a low dose of amitriptyline, twenty-five milligrams. You're nowhere near the ceiling. It's your call."

"Since my amitriptyline dose is low, I should be okay, right?" I tried to think through the decision, but my brain kept stumbling. It had become hard to think since I started the ECT. "Yeah, I'll take it. I can't even wear close-toed shoes because my toes hurt so bad from this."

Kelly had handed me a prescription for terbinafine.

Twice a week, Andrew drove us to Local Hospital. He sat with his iPad and bathed in the soft rays of sunrise while Dr. Iyilik or Dr. Pintalabios shocked my brain. I couldn't tell if the treatments were helping, because I slept the entire day after each one.

During the rare times I was awake, I'd hear music that wasn't there. Well, not really music, more like clusters of tones that sounded musical. Sometimes it sounded like monks chanting or voices singing—not that I could make out any words. Other times it was a bunch of notes together in quick succession, like a Thelonious Monk composition. And it was constant. If I was conscious, the sounds were playing in my head.

I thought about going to an audiologist to get checked out, but I figured that once the audiologist found out I was having ECT, they'd decide I was just having crazy-person hallucinations and send me back to Dr. Iyilik. So, I didn't bother with audiology. Dr. Iyilik knew about the music already. I'd told him and Becky, the ECT nurse about it, and they'd just been like, "Huh. Okay. No idea what that is. How's your mood?"

"Terrible. I still want to die every month until my period starts. I don't even want to have a baby anymore. I'm too sick to be a parent. I don't know what I was thinking," I answered Dr. Iyilik.

"Well, since you aren't trying for a baby anymore, we can try a more powerful antidepressant. Let's move you off the Viibryd Dr. Boatbill had you on and start you on a low dose of amitriptyline," he suggested.

"Okay," I murmured.

I spoke again, "I can't remember anything from minute to minute. I put my dogs in the backyard and then forget to let them back in until I hear them barking an hour later. I put water on for tea, and two minutes later I freak out at the sound of the boiling water because I've forgotten I turned the teapot on. Maybe I should stop the ECT. I don't like this. It's scaring me."

"Short-term memory loss is a normal short-term side effect of ECT. It will go away in a few weeks—a month or two at most. That's what the studies say," he assured me.

Against my better judgment, I trusted him.

~~

"I'm still doing ECT at Local Hospital, but it's not helping at all with the PMDD. It's just making me sleep all day and destroying my memory," I reported at my next appointment with Dr. Fahrig.

"PMDD gets worse with age," she said. "That's what I've seen in my practice and heard from my colleagues. I'm not surprised that it's gotten this bad over time.

"Oral birth control isn't showing the benefit I'd hoped for," she continued. "We can try an injection called Lupron. Lupron will activate a state of chemically induced menopause. That should stop all of your PMDD symptoms."

"Seriously?" I asked. "All of them will stop with a shot? Let's do it."

Andrew was more prudent. "What are the potential side effects? Twilah seems very prone to adverse reactions."

"It can cause hot flashes and hair loss in some women," Dr. Fahrig warned. "With long-term use, it can have more serious side effects, like loss of bone density, so I won't be able to prescribe it for more than six months. But short term should be fine."

*Hot flashes and hair loss versus a monthly drive to die?* "Yes, I'd like to try the Lupron please," I said.

In May 2014, Dr. Iyilik cut the ECT from twice weekly to once every other week. Now that I could stay awake for more than four hours at a time, I looked for another job. I accepted a position as a department manager at a natural foods store. I packed for the trip to Colorado where I'd undergo training for my new position.

On June 20, 2014, I got my first Lupron injection. Nine days later, I boarded a plane to Denver. When I arrived, I picked up my rental car and dug the directions I'd printed out of my purse. I used the navigation on my iPhone for backup though I preferred visual directions to Siri's voice.

I spent the next four hours circling Denver. My destination was a hotel in a town called Broomfield. Locating Broomfield was impossible. I could no longer read the print on the paper I held. The directions had collapsed into a meaningless jumble of letters. The voice of the iPhone was similarly indecipherable.

"Ache exiii blahhhhhhh, continue on hahway blahhhhhhh," said Siri.

I passed the same landmarks again and again. My eyes couldn't focus. The letters on road signs bounced and blurred.

"Call Andrew," I said to Siri. "I'm lost. I, I, I can't find Broomfield!" I cried when Andrew picked up.

"Didn't blah oooh take directions?" Andrew asked.

"Y-yes! But, I can't read them. I'm lost!" I repeated.

Andrew seemed annoyed but helped me navigate to the hotel. I struggled to understand his voice, but when I plugged in my earbuds and listened through them, it became easier to decode his speech.

I arrived at the hotel. I hung back near the entrance while a family with several small children checked in before me. The lobby looked abnormally large. The walls leaned in toward me. I tapped my foot gingerly in front of me to orient myself in the space. After I checked in, I stumbled up the stairs to my room. I lay down on the bed and watched my thoughts race through my mind, disjointed and chaotic. I breathed deeply and tried to meditate, but I couldn't achieve clarity. Jumbled illuminated letters flashed through my head.

I awoke to heavy bleeding. Dr. Fahrig hadn't told me I'd have a period after the injection. I stumbled down the stairs and gazed at the small shelf of toiletries displayed in the lobby. The packages seemed to lean and ooze into one another.

"Can I help you?"

I jumped at the sound of the clerk's voice.

My eyes turned to the carpet under my feet as I froze. I needed tampons, but I was terrified of this man.

"Uh, uh, uh. Where can I get like, uh, lady stuff?"

"There's a Blah-Mart two blocks away. You just blah. Go blah. Down blah." He pointed toward the parking lot.

After circling for twenty minutes, I located the store and bought my necessities. Then I set out for the training facility in Golden. I somehow managed to find it on my first try.

The trainers handed each of the new managers a folder filled with onboarding material. Like the directions I'd printed, the handouts were filled with letters that lay toppled in a pile. I tried to listen to the trainers, but their speech was blurred and indistinct, far more so than speech had been my entire life. I stared at my computer screen and tried to submit an order for the eighth time. The rest of the class had moved to the next exercise ten minutes prior. I took a breath and tried again. *ERROR*, the dancing letters on the screen flashed as my eyes rushed to chase them down.

I stood and ran to the bathroom. I blinked back tears and told myself to breathe. *Why can't I read? Why can't I hear? What's happening to me?* Panic rose in my chest, but I redirected my thoughts. *It'll be okay. Job training has always been confusing.*

I returned to the classroom and stared at the computer.

"Finish that later." A trainer had appeared beside me and was speaking into my ear. "Don't hold up the class." When I finally figured out what she'd said, my face reddened.

After class, I took several wrong turns on the drive back to Broomfield. *This dusty country highway looks like a good place to die.* I pushed the thought away and drove in circles and meanders until I found the hotel. I put my earbuds in and called Andrew.

"Oh my God, I don't know what's happening to me! I can't think! I'm so confused."

"What do you mean, honey? What's happening? You've always have a hard time with job training, but you always catch on eventually," he assured me.

"No, it's not my normal trouble. It's different. I don't know, I'm just confused. I can't think. My brain isn't working!"

"Do you need me to come out there? I can be there in nine hours."

"No, no, I'll keep trying. I'm just confused," I insisted. "Confused. Confused. Confused. Confuso, confusee, confusee, confooooo!" I chanted as the ends of the words seemed to pull from my mouth like taffy. "Ima, Ima, Ima justa meditate more and work on my concentration. Yep, yep, yep!"

Andrew's concern had bolstered my ebbing determination.

"I've had harder jobs, jobs. I'll figure this out, out, out," I said before ending the call.

The next morning, I got lost driving to Golden. I lowered my eyes as I walked into the classroom twenty minutes late.

That afternoon, the trainers taught us how to operate the cash registers. The exercise took place on a simulated sales floor, complete with music that played from speakers overhead. The music poured into my ears and chopped up my thoughts. Beep! Beep! Beep! The sound of the scanner sent red javelins of pain through my head.

After an hour on the registers, a trainer named Pam took us to another room. "As blah as you count down blah cash drawers, we can wrap up blah today," she said. I couldn't understand her, so I watched my coworkers to figure out what we'd been told to do.

I tried to hide my tears as I counted the bills over and over. Each time, I arrived at a different figure, none of which were correct. I was the last trainee left in the room.

"Are you blah trouble with yours? You just blah to count it down to fifty blah," Pam said.

"I, Ima, Ima. I keep getting different numbers. I don't know why." Tears welled up. I dropped the Monopoly money onto the table and ran to the parking lot.

I found my way back to the hotel and left a voicemail for my human resources liaison.

"Um, hi, Lisa. This is Twilah Hiari, and I'm out here training for the body care manager position at the new Kansas store. Um, something's wrong. I'm sick. Ima, Ima, um, having problems, problems, problems, thinking. I need to go home now. I'm really sorry, sorry, sorry, but please, please, get me a fly birdo home."

Two hours later, the phone rang. "Hi, Twilah. I got blah-blah message. What's going blah? Is blah-blah altitude?" she asked. "Lots of trainees get altitude sickness. We'd be happy blah-blah medical treatment for that."

"What?" I couldn't understand her. She'd called the hotel phone, and I couldn't plug in my earbuds.

She repeated her question about altitude sickness. "No, no, it's not the altitude. It's something else. Please, Ima, Ima, needa go home," I pleaded.

"We can get blah to a doctor here and blah you checked out."

"Just get me a fucking flight!" I dropped the phone, stunned by my anger. I hadn't had an outburst like this since I'd stop taking Prozac.

I closed my eyes until the phone rang again. "Twilah, this blah Lisa again. I emailed blah flight information. Do blah me to order a cab blah to drive to the airport?"

She repeated her question until I finally understood. "Yes, yes, yes. Ima, cab please. Cab, cab, cab, please!" I begged.

Two and a half hours later, I was walking my third lap around the Denver airport. The walls leaned in toward me, and the ceiling pulsed like a beating heart.

"You gotta blah go through the line blah again. You can't blah laptop in carryon. Blah it out." The woman in the black uniform had taken my bag. I had no idea what was happening.

"Bay meep laptop fly home me now say?" I asked.

The TSA attendant stared. I stumbled through the rest of security, certain I'd be arrested at any time.

Andrew picked me up from the airport. At home, I curled up with my dogs and slept for two days straight.

༄

***How was your difficulty in this training different from your previous challenges in training environments?***

Well, it was like what I'd experienced before, but amplified by about a hundred times. And I'd worked in a grocery store from 1994 to 1999. I'd worked in lots of different departments, including as a cashier. And I'd never been bothered by the music that played overhead. It'd never interfered with my ability to count money or do anything else. But the music completely destroyed my focus in Colorado. I couldn't block it out. That had never been a problem before.

# CHAPTER SIXTEEN

MY HEART WAS a big thumping creature, a giant rabbit forcing its legs against my chest wall. I could hear the blood pushing past my jaw and surging into my forehead. *Whoosh, whoosh, thump.* I could hear all the organs in my body, and at the same time I could hear even the tiniest little sounds in the environment around me. I recognized neither my mind nor the world I inhabited.

I woke from a turbulent sleep. My clothing and the mattress beneath me were soaked in sweat. My brain was a balloon inflated beyond capacity. I opened my eyes and gritted my teeth. The pressure inside my skull was unbearable. I pushed myself onto my knees. I pulled back like a rattlesnake before propelling my forehead into the wall.

Andrew rushed over to me. "What are you doing?" he yelled as I launched my head against the wall again.

"Smash. Smash. Smash. Ima gotta smash." Tears streamed down my face as I slammed my head against the wall.

"What blah hell? Stop it! Oh my God, Twilah! Go back blah

sleep." He'd wrapped his arms around me and pulled me away from the wall.

When he went back to sleep, I snuck over to his nightstand. I reached into the drawer and pulled out several bottles. I peered at the labels, but the letters blurred together. I shook several pills into my hands and shoved them into my mouth.

Andrew woke up. "Oh my God! Blah are blah doing?"

Minutes later, we were at Local Hospital.

"You tried to overdose!" shouted the ER nurse. I stared at his mouth to augment my understanding of his words.

"Yeah, meep," I murmured.

"What did you take?" he asked.

"I don't know. Bay! Just medicine from the drawer. Meep! Some Ativan maybe, and Ima don't know, some painkillers—mmmmm—" My words collapsed into a low buzz.

"If you took Ativan, why don't your labs show benzodiazepines?" he challenged.

"Huh?" I looked to Andrew for help. I didn't know how lab tests worked. But my husband's narrowed eyes were aimed at the nurse. I could feel rage radiating from both men.

The nurse stalked out of the room, muttering something that sounded like a little like "drug seeker."

I didn't want to be in this hospital again. I didn't want to be on this earth anymore. But upstairs I went.

I looked at my wristband for my assigned psychiatrist's name. I sorted through the blurred and dancing letters—*Dr. Thueban.*

Dr. Thueban came to my room early the next morning. He was an attractive man with dark-green eyes. He looked to be about my age. He had thick, loose waves of hair and copper-colored skin. He crossed his legs and regarded me.

"Why blah you blah overdose?" he asked. His vaguely Middle Eastern accent seemed to propel the words from his mouth at an unusually rapid rate. After asking for repetition several times, I tried to answer him.

"I'm really confused, and I'm having horrible anxiety. Nothing makes sense. I can barely s-s-s-say the words I'm trying to say. MEEP!" I continued, "I went to Colorado t-t-to train for a job. But I couldn't do anything out there. I'm so confused. I couldn't count money or anything! Something's wrong. Nothing makes sense. M-m-math has never been my strong suit, but I'm a college graduate, I can do f-f-freaking basic arithmetic. Or I could before. I can't now. Can't count. Can't count! I'm so confused—"

"I see you have a history of depression," he said as he flipped through some papers.

"Yes, yes. But that's not why I'm here now. Now, now, now. I'm not depressed. Ima, Ima, Ima confused. Confused. And anxious. Anxious. And t-t-tired. And mixed up. I tried to die because I can't think, and I want to smash my head. Smash, smash! Meep—I'm not supposed to smash. No smash, no smash! I'm so confused—"

"And PTSD?" he went on as though I hadn't spoken.

"Huh? Uh-huh."

"Do you have nightmares?"

"Yes."

"Tell me about them," he said softly.

I stared into my mind and tried to organize my thoughts. "Last night, I dreamed that my husband got tired of me being sick, sick. Ima dreamed he l-l-left meeeeeeep! MEEP!" I screamed.

"I see." He nodded. "Well, to start, let's get you on a therapeutic dose of amitriptyline. You're on a very low dose of twenty-five milligrams. Let's increase that."

"Okaaay," I slurred. He closed his folder and stood.

"I will come see you again tomorrow," he said.

"Okaaay," I repeated. Seconds later, I was asleep.

When I woke up, my stomach felt contorted. After forty-five minutes of painful diarrhea, I left my room and found a nurse.

"Ima, Ima been fighting C. diff on and off s-since April or May, and I think it's b-b-back," I said.

The young man's eyes widened. "Let me look at your stool," Nurse Ratched demanded.

I ran to the bathroom and expelled another rancid pile. Blisters formed on my skin everywhere the diarrhea touched it.

"That is not C. diff!" he declared after peering at the mass in the toilet.

"Don't you need a lab t-test to tell you th-th-that?" I asked.

"No, I don't. I'm a *nurse*, and I know C. diff. C. diff is a very bad infection. You don't have C. diff. You have anxiety." He rolled his eyes.

Over the next four days, Dr. Thueban increased my amitriptyline dosage from twenty-five milligrams to 150 milligrams.

"How did you sleep?" Dr. Thueban asked.

"I didn't! It was terrible! My l-l-legs wouldn't stop moving—I'm so confused, confused—meep—I can't think!" I started.

"Yes, yes, yes—but how is your mood?" Dr. Thueban interrupted.

"Okay. I'm just tired and confused."

"Are you having any more thoughts of harming yourself?"

"Noooo! Meep. Bay!"

"Okay, then you can go home today."

"Okaaay."

Andrew picked me up and drove me straight to his lab. A fresh analysis revealed I had C. diff again.

I called Local Hospital. "Um, meeep, hi. May Ima, Ima speak to the director of nursing, um p-please?"

"She's not available. I can take a message and have her call you back," the woman who'd answered the phone offered.

After several whats and huhs, I understood her. "Ima, Ima just c-c-calling to meep say I just um learned that I had C. diff when I was there last week. Ima thought um, meep, you should know to clean the room I stayed in especially w-w-well."

"Oh! Thank you for calling us about that. I'll make sure the director calls you back!" the woman exclaimed.

The call never came.

Meanwhile, I struggled to read the dancing words on my discharge paperwork.

*Borderline personality disorder,*
*Post-traumatic stress disorder,*

*Major depressive disorder, recurrent, severe without psychotic features*
*Generalized anxiety disorder*

Andrew took me back to Local Hospital and we got the rest of my records for the stay.

**History of Present Illness:**
The patient presents with severe worsening of depression over the last month. She indicates depressed mood, anhedonia, hopelessness, helplessness, decreased self-esteem, decreased energy, and frequent thoughts of suicide with a plan to overdose on medications. She experienced significant stress after attempting to get a job in Colorado. She returned home within 2 days due to feeling overwhelmed. She denies mania or psychosis, no homicidal ideation. She denies substance misuse.

**Past Psychiatric History:**
The patient has numerous psychiatric hospitalizations. This is the second hospitalization this year and 6 within the last 7 years. She started having thoughts of suicide at age 8 when she tried to hang herself in her closet. She also had attempts to overdose and cut her wrist starting at age 13. She denies a history of substance misuse. She has been tried on numerous medications in the past including Prozac, Paxil, Celexa, Lexapro, Effexor, Cymbalta, Remeron, Viibryd, Wellbutrin, amitriptyline, prazosin, and Deplin. She indicates a history of emotional and physical abuse and re-experiencing symptoms and anxiety related to that. She has been receiving electroconvulsive therapy for the last 2 months and a half under the care of Dr. Iyilik.

**Family History:**
Significant for both mental illness and addiction. No known family history of suicide.

**Social History:**
The patient is a 38-year-old white female. She is married to her husband of 7 years. No children. She has a bachelor degree level of education. She has been unemployed for the last 14 years due to psychiatric disability.

**Past Medical History:**
The patient is physically healthy.

**Laboratory Data:**
CBC [complete blood count] within normal limits. BMP [basic metabolic panel] within normal limits. LFTs [liver function tests] slightly elevated . . . Toxicology screen was negative . . .

**Mental Status Examination:**
The patient is a 38-year-old white female appearing her stated age with fair grooming and hygiene. She was alert and oriented x3. She exhibits mild psychomotor agitation. She was somewhat uncooperative, refusing to attend groups. She was depressed with labile, tearful affect. She has clear sensorium with no auditory or visual hallucinations. No delusions were noted. Thought process was linear and goal directed. She continues to have thoughts of suicide. No homicidal ideation. Severely impaired insight and impaired judgment.

**7/11/2014**
PATIENT TOLERATED INCREASED Amitriptyline. SHE REPORTS FEELING LESS DEPRESSED. SHE HAS LESS FREQUENT THOUGHTS OF DYING "ONLY ONCE SINCE THIS MORNING." SHE CONTINUES TO BE WITHDRAWN, ISOLATING HERSELF IN HER ROOM AND REFUSING GROUPS. I DISCUSSED HER CARE IN A TEAM MEETING. WE'LL INCREASE Amitriptyline TO A THERAPEUTIC DOSE.

07/12/2014

PATIENT REPORTS MODERATE SEDATION WITH INCREASED DOSE OF Amitriptyline. STILL, SHE NOTES IMPROVED MOOD OVERALL. NO S/I TODAY. WE'LL SWITCH Amitriptyline DOSING TO BEDTIME.

07/13/2014

Patient notes improved mood. No S/H/I [suicidal/homicidal ideation]. More than thirty minutes were spent on discharge day.

The hospitalization had been my third, not second, of the year. My "mild psychomotor agitation" had been the first sign of an abnormal mouth movement or tic that would persist for almost two years. The movement consisted of the drawing down of the lower left side of my mouth. Among neurologists, this is known as an extrapyramidal movement. It's a feature of drug-induced movement disorders.

I hadn't been unemployed for fourteen years. I'd been unemployed for three days, and prior to that I hadn't been employed full-time for fifteen months. I'd worked each Saturday in the summer helping out at the farmers market. I'd taken breaks from that job each time the C. diff had come back. Now, I couldn't return since I'd lost my ability to count money.

*Nurse Ratched didn't want to consider that you had C. diff, and Dr. Thueban didn't want to consider that you might be having an adverse reaction to amitriptyline, Lupron, ECT, or anything else.*

Huh? What? Was that even a question? Let me get through all those words—well, of course. It's the whole credibility thing again. I had none. There's a term that describes when a patient is presumed to be crazy and the doctor attributes every symptom or complaint to the patient's perceived psychiatric condition. It's called *diagnostic overshadowing*. But I call it *being an incompetent asshole*.

The C. diff issue though, that got interesting. After my run-in with Ratched, I'd called Andrew. Andrew had come to the hospital and demanded to speak to Ratched's supervisor. After that meeting, Ratched agreed to send my sample down to the lab. But the lab rejected the sample, and Andrew threw his hands up. Funny thing though, in 2016, Andrew was in a citywide lab meeting, and Local Hospital's lab manager was there. Andrew brought up the incident to him. The lab manager said he'd talk to his microbiology people, and they'd reconsider their processes.

But how messed up is that—that you need that kind of *in* to the system, that kind of clout, to get things done properly?

∽

"Dr. Thueban said I have b-b-borderline personality disorder," I explained.

Dr. Iyilik shook his head. "That's news to me," he said.

"I don't think it's right. I read about it, and I don't think I m-m-meet the criteria. I don't think it's right that he wrote that in my r-r-records. Meep! Meep!"

"You don't meet the criteria," Dr. Iyilik agreed. He sat back and appeared to be thinking. "I can talk to him, and you can request that the record be changed. It doesn't happen often, but it can be done."

"I w-will. Bay!"

Dr. Iyilik continued to look at me. "Have you noticed a difference in your speech?" he asked.

"Y-y-yeah. My words are c-c-coming out all j-j-jumbled. I can't t-t-think either." Tears welled. "I, I, I'm so confused. Meep!"

Dr. Iyilik's eyes seemed to reflect the concern I felt. "Have you noticed that your mouth is drawing down a bit?"

"Y-y-yeah, that too," I moaned.

"Maybe it's the Lupron? I don't know, but I think you should see a neurologist. Call this doctor. His name is Dr. Wise, and he's very, very good. Please. Call him right away." He scrolled through his tablet and wrote a phone number on a piece of paper.

At the check-out desk, I struggled to write my follow-up appointment date in my planner. My hand couldn't force the pen to form the letters, and I couldn't tell how much space I had on the paper to fit the words. I made some indecipherable squiggles then gave up and asked for a reminder card.

I paced the parking lot for several minutes before I located my car. Then I got lost on the drive home. I'd been to Dr. Iyilik's office many times before. It was only a few miles from my house. I circled in unfamiliar neighborhoods until I located major streets. Once I found the major streets, I guessed at the direction I should point my car. I could no longer identify my location on the planet.

At home, I squinted at my iPhone and tapped out the number Dr. Iyilik had given me. The call rolled straight to voicemail.

"Um, hi, my name is T-W-I-L-A-H, H-I-A-R-I. Ima, Ima c-c-calling to schedule an appointment w-w-with Dr. Wise. Please c-c-call me back," I said, then gave my phone number. "Meep." I pressed end.

*Ring!* My phone blared several hours later. I aimed my finger at the green icon and missed as the ringing continued. I finally caught the icon as it was falling off the edge of the screen. "H-hello? Meep!"

"This is Blahhhhh from Blah-er Blah-ise office, you blah-all blah-pointment?"

I paused to sort through the sounds.

"Hello!" she blasted.

"Uh, this is Twilah Hiari. I'd called for an a-a-appointment with Dr. W-W-Wise."

"Well, what do y-blah need the ap-blah-ment? You need a blah G?" she blurted out an acronym that I couldn't decipher. "Or a blah-blah."

"Huh?"

"What's yer diagnosis? Why blah you eed to ee Dr. Wise!" She was shouting now.

"I, I, I don't have a d-d-diag—"

"I need your diagnosis!" she yelled.

I slapped the red end icon with my palm before squinting at the phone and tapping out a text to Andrew. *Would you please call Dr. Wise's office and get me an appointment?* It took me several minutes to construct the message.

---

On August 7, I was back at Dr. Fahrig's office. "This is for any updates," said the receptionist as she pushed a clipboard across the desk.

I leaned down to hear her words, then took the clipboard and found a seat in the waiting area. I gazed at the top sheet and watched the ink ooze off of the paper. My eyes scanned up and down, but nothing I did could freeze the letters in place before they spilled off the page. A television planted on the waiting room wall blared, and the sound tore across my brain.

"P-p-please do this." I handed the clipboard to Andrew. A minute later, we were called back to a treatment room.

As soon as Dr. Fahrig entered, her usual cheery expression turned to one of concern.

"How've you been doing?" she asked tentatively.

"N-n-not—good. I'm really um, confused. Meep. But my m-m-mood is better."

Dr. Fahrig stared. "How much amitriptyline are you on?"

"One hundred fifty muh-uh-uh—" I looked to Andrew for help.

"One hundred fifty milligrams," he responded. "Her mood's way better since the Lupron, but she's really confused, and her speech is seriously impaired. Is it possible the Lupron's doing this?"

"I don't think it's the Lupron. It's more likely the amitriptyline. You should see a neurologist right away. Your speech is very distorted, and your mouth movement is very unusual."

I looked at her but couldn't speak. I peered into my mind at where the words I wanted to say usually appeared, but I only saw blazes of rainbow light.

"That's what Dr. Iyilik told her to do—see a neurologist. Dr. Iyilik's never seen anything like this," Andrew said.

Dr. Fahrig continued to regard me. "You might ask Dr. Iyilik if he can lower your dose of amitriptyline. Do you have a neurology appointment yet?"

"Huh? Uh. Meep. Bay!" I looked at Andrew.

"Yes, she's scheduled to see Dr. Wise later this month. That's who Dr. Iyilik recommended. Do you know him?"

"No, I don't know him. But it's good that you're scheduled," she said. She paused before speaking again.

"Well, I'm glad your mood is improved. We'll continue the Lupron injections. Please let me know what the neurologist says. Do you still have the C. diff?"

I opened and closed my mouth but could form no speech. I looked to my husband.

"Yes," Andrew answered. "She's seeing a gastroenterologist for it. She's had several rounds of vancomycin and several rounds of Dificid, but it keeps coming back."

Dr. Fahrig nodded solemnly. "Please keep me updated."

I nodded and took a sip from my water bottle. My mouth had become so dry that each word I managed to unleash was accompanied by loud sucking and smacking sounds.

I lapsed into exhaustion as my sleep became more disturbed. I'd wake throughout the night to the sensation of constant kicking. My legs thrusted and jerked with an impulse and urgency I couldn't curb.

*You can obviously read now. How long did it take you to get that skill back?*

I can't remember. I still can't read as easily as I used to though. I just can't concentrate. And I still have intermittent visual problems. They come in episodes after I eat anything starchy or sweet or citrusy, or when I'm having an allergic reaction to anything. I get a kind of warning because the pitch and volume of my tinnitus changes. But even when I'm not having an allergic reaction, I can't stand for anything to move when I'm trying to read. Things like GIFs destroy my ability to focus because my cognitive relationship to movement has changed. If there's motion around text, I can't read at all. I never had that problem before 2014.

# CHAPTER SEVENTEEN

I'D KNOWN MY stylist for about six years. I'd always hated haircuts, but my familiarity with Shawna made the process tolerable.

The music from the speakers embedded in the ceiling of the salon was like lightning strikes to my cerebral cortex. My eyes were drawn to a flash of movement. I turned my head and saw that Shawna was waving at me. My eyes fixated on the motion of her hand. "Blah-as-blah go-blah-on," she yelled. "You blah-oo-blah like a blah-eaker."

"Huh?" I forced my eyes to her mouth as she repeated the sentence.

"You're doing that chewing thing like a tweaker. You know, a meth head?"

My jaw was rotating. I couldn't make it stop. I sorted through her words. I sat silently as she cut my hair. In the mirror, I watched my jaw perform its circumambulations. Tears puddled at the corners of my eyes.

"You've got some bald patches, girl. Like somebody on chemo. Are you okay?" Shawna asked. I stared at her lips in the mirror and slowly absorbed her words. I shrugged in return. Words wouldn't form in my mind or mouth.

That night, Andrew drove us to a shoe store.

"These shoes, shoes, foots, um, bay! Shoes, meep!" I blurted at the salesman. I shook my head and saw orbs of light. I finished the transaction by scratching words onto my notepad. The salesman struggled to decipher the malformed letters I'd created on the page.

As we neared home, my arms became numb. My jaw continued to rotate like a motorized hinge. Andrew drove to the emergency room of Local Hospital. The staff rushed me back for treatment because of my strokelike symptoms.

A nurse with long, bright-pink acrylic nails looked down at me. I lay on a bed beneath her gaze. "What's happening, hon?" she asked. I stared at the floral designs on her fingertips. I struggled to understand her, then tried to answer her question. "I, uh, uh, I, uh." I stammered out stunted sounds, then took my notepad out of my purse and tried to write.

"Do you use sign language?" she asked. "We can get you an interpreter."

"No!" Andrew yelled. "That's why we're here! She's not deaf. She knows how to speak, but she can't right now."

"Oh, she sounded deaf—" The nurse tapped her claws on a clipboard, and the sound echoed in my head.

"Her speech has been getting worse for weeks, and now it's gone! This is because of the amitriptyline or the Lupron. She got a second Lupron shot a couple of days ago," Andrew said.

The doctor, a young man with short blond hair, strode into the room. "What's going on?" he asked. Despite his unaccented Midwestern English, he was hard to understand. I struggled to hear him over the beeping instruments around me.

I scribbled on my notepad.

"No!" he shouted. "I want you to tell me! Use your words!"

I opened my mouth. "Muh-muh-meep! MEEP! Bay! Bay!" Bright letters danced in my field of vision. A choir roared in my left ear, and a bee buzzed steadily in my right ear.

The floor shook beneath me as a man pushed my bed down the hall for a CT scan. Minutes later, he wheeled me back to the original room.

The young doctor shook the piece of paper in his hand. "Your CT blah normal! This cannot blah the amitriptyline," he declared. "I've never seen a drug reaction blah this. Blah-blah. Conversion disorder! I saw your psychiatric history! You're converting blah stress into physical symptoms."

His expression was that of a man who'd just found dog shit on his shoe.

"I'm going to give you blah Ativan. Follow up with blah psychiatrist," he said before stalking from the room.

I tried to say I didn't want the Ativan. Ativan always made me want to die. But I couldn't speak, and no one was listening. Acrylic Nurse pumped Ativan into my IV.

*What's the difference in your loss of speech in this time period versus how you hadn't been able to talk before in meetings or therapy?*

The difference is before, I could form thoughts and words in my mind, but I was scared to speak or couldn't figure out when to speak. It was an anxiety and timing thing. And it only happened in certain situations. I've always been able to communicate very well when I'm one on one with the few people who are close to me. This time I could neither form thoughts nor get my words out. It had nothing to do with anxiety. There'd been a complete disengagement of the communication components within my brain.

*Do you think if you didn't have a psych history the ER doctor would've been more objective?*

Hell yeah, I do. I'm not saying he would have correctly diagnosed me. He wouldn't have. He didn't have the knowledge or the resources. But he probably wouldn't have treated me like dog shit, no.

And his hubris! Astonishing, isn't it? I mean, he said, "I've never seen a drug reaction like this." And that somehow translated to, "I couldn't be having a drug reaction." Because if he—this little boy doctor, in this little Kansas hospital, hasn't seen something—then it can't exist? Are you fucking kidding me? Do you think he knew that Lupron has a rare but known side effect of pituitary apoplexy? Do you think he knew that amitriptyline can cause something called neuroleptic malignant syndrome? Do you think he had a comprehensive pharmaceutical side-effect database in his teeny little head? Of course he didn't!

But even though he didn't have knowledge, he had power—the power to brand me with the ultimate crazy bitch diagnosis of conversion disorder. You know, it's one thing to make a diagnostic mistake based on inadequate information—but it's an entirely different thing to blame the patient for your mistake, treat them like shit for it, and destroy their reputation through their medical record.

This was a turning point. It's when I realized that biases are more dangerous than I'd ever imagined, because once enough authorities canonize a bias as truth, you're screwed.

**What do you mean?**

Huh? What do I mean? I'll try to explain. It's a manipulation that seems logical on the face of it if you don't know what to look for. You know what a syllogism is, right? No? Well, bear with me. It's not that hard.

A syllogism is a form of reasoning where you have a major premise, a minor premise, and a conclusion. That's the bare bones basics, and that's all you need to know right now. I'm gonna use a particular syllogism called Modus Felapton here.

**You said particular syllogism? How many syllogisms are there?**

Huh? How many? Twenty-four valid ones, but 256 in total. Stop interrupting me! You want me to get all circus sideshow autistic and name all the syllogisms? No, thank you.

Anyway, one syllogism that has a special appeal to doctors goes like this: No mentally ill person is worthy of decent treatment from me. All mentally ill people are without easily detectible organic causes for their unconventional behavior. Some mentally ill people exist. Therefore, some people without easily detectable organic causes for their behavior are not worthy of decent treatment from me.

It's easy for an emotionally motivated, egotistical doctor to see this syllogism as valid. I mean, it sounds good, right? Of course, once you adopt this line of thinking, all hope for offering fair treatment to a patient who presents as mentally ill is gone.

Now, there are a lot of things wrong with that syllogism. But do you think that most emotionally motivated egomaniacs will see the problems? I don't. Let me point out just a few issues. First, if any of your premises are false, the whole thing falls apart. And we have reason to question both premises. Do you see the odd concept here, the concept of a different character? No?

Worthy of decent treatment, that's the concept, and it's a real tricky one. It probably doesn't belong in this format, but would you have recognized that if I hadn't told you? Do you understand why *worthy of decent treatment* is different? Why it doesn't fit in? Of course you don't, because you're more emotional than you are rational. But I see instantly that the concepts *worthy* and *decent* are different from the types of concepts you usually see in valid syllogisms. They're vague, and they rest on a lot of moral assumptions.

And then there's what's known as the problem of the empty class, which leads to what's known as an existential fallacy. You're lost? Hold on, chill out, this isn't hard. All the empty class means is that you're referring to something that isn't there. The classic example is saying all unicorns have one horn. There are no unicorns, so it doesn't matter what qualities, like the number of horns, they have. The unicorn class is empty.

What if there are no mentally ill people? What if mental illness is an empty class? I mean, unless you're ready to explain how all these behaviors, which can vary from time period to time period and circumstance to circumstance, are enduring enough to be considered qualities, like the quality of redness or the quality of having a horn—or even like the quality of having heart disease or diabetes—then your *Diagnostic and Statistical Manual of Mental Disorders* is starting to look like a big book of unicorn breed descriptions. You should call it *The Unicorn Almanac,* not the DSM! Or should you? Am I trying to trick you? Can you even tell? Do you feel manipulated? Deceived? Screwed and confused? That's how I felt when I read my medical records—like I'd been tricked. Like the doctors had used something that they were supposed to have professional mastery of and turned around and fucked me with it.

So back to the syllogism. Since you can't identify the problems in the example, you're probably at risk for believing something that looks valid but isn't valid at all. There are lots of problems with that example, but the logical form is legit.

And there I was with unconventional behavior and no easily detectable organic cause. The doctor concluded I was mentally ill, and therefore unworthy of decent treatment.

# CHAPTER EIGHTEEN

I STARED OUT the passenger-side window at the giant oak trees. Their branches waved like the axes of executioners. I pressed myself into the seat and drew my knees to my chest. It was late August, and the hot, humid Kansas summer was drawing to a close. I wondered if my brain would make it through another season.

The doctor gently closed the door to the exam room. My eyes took in his wispy white hair.

"Hello, blah Dr. Wise. Blah brings blah here today?" he asked.

"Uh, um, Ima, uh—I started getting confused meep when I was having ECT earlier um, uh, this year. Then, um, I s-s-started to have um, problems w-w-with my memory. Then um this doctor um in-in-increased my ami-ami-ami—" I stuttered for a moment before Andrew interjected and offered a more concise report of the events. Occasionally, I inserted a sentence or two into his narrative.

"Oh, and I, uh, saw—um, online that terbinafine and uh, amitriptyline are um contraindicated and I—BAY! I was um, taking t-terbinafine at the s-s-ame time this happened. Meep!"

"What else did you find in your Googling?" Dr. Wise shot back.

I closed my mouth. He'd interrupted me. I took a breath and tried to change direction, but no more words came. I opened and closed my mouth a few more times but couldn't create speech.

Wise led me through a series of exercises. I extended my arm and reached back to touch my nose. I ambled down the hallway and back as he watched. I struggled to follow his instructions but managed to do as he asked.

"What all psychiatric drugs blah you taken?" he asked.

"L-l-like ever?"

"Yes, blah the course of blah whole life."

I looked to Andrew, who rattled off a comprehensive list.

"This is *not* conversion disorder," Dr. Wise stated. His voice was firm. "This is tardive dyskinesia. Stop the amitriptyline. Avoid blah antiemetics, anticholinergics, and neuroleptic blah if possible. Since your exposure to blah high dose of amitriptyline was of a relatively short duration, this may go blah in time."

After I'd fought to understand his words, I'd struggled to ask how the relatively sudden onset of my symptoms meshed with a diagnosis of tardive dyskinesia. I hadn't heard the term before, but the Latin root was clear. Tardive would mean late, not sudden or acute.

"You've been blah psychiatric medications for years. Over time, those medications, especially antipsychotics blah Seroquel and Abilify, can create the conditions blah make changes like this possible," he said.

I nodded as I sorted through his words.

"Oo-kay," I said. He stood and extended his hand. I shook it and followed Andrew out the door.

I left the appointment feeling both relieved and concerned. Relieved that Dr. Wise had said my symptoms might resolve, but I was concerned that I'd never been warned this could happen. Not a single psychiatrist had advised me of this potential outcome. Dr. Pintalabios had prescribed Seroquel, and Dr. Boatbill had been giving me Abilify samples for years.

Weeks later, I read Dr. Wise's report.

> On an outpatient basis (after discharge by Thueban), she noticed the appearance of a number of symptoms that progressively worsened over the ensuing days. They included impaired concentration, difficulty reading and speaking, and problems finding appropriate words. Her balance and walking were "slow, not my normal pace," and she became extremely sensitive to noise. Visual hallucinations occurred on one occasion. It was unclear regarding auditory. At some point, involuntary movements began as well and included jaw jutting, back and forth movement of the lower jaw and tongue protrusions . . . These involuntary movements increased to the point that she was "mute, nonverbal." . . . On about 08/04/14, she was lethargic, lacked focus, lacked energy. Could not do her daily routine. She was forgetful including how to sew, an activity she has done on a regular basis. She and her husband Googled the interaction of LAMISIL and AMITRIPTYLINE and noted that LAMISIL inhibits the hepatic enzyme, CYP2D6, which is an important intermediate enzyme in the metabolism of AMITRIPTYLINE to NORTRIPTYLINE. Consequently, the amount of AMITRIPTYLINE in the blood can increase and produce central nervous system side effects. The medication was discontinued.

That was all accurate. But when I read his note under my diagnosis of major depression, recurrent, chronic, I was struck by what seemed to be inevitable disappointment.

> As noted by multiple psychiatrists, it [major depression] is severe with suicidal impulse. It appears refractory to treatment. I do not believe there was any intent to cause harm when the dismissal medications were prescribed as they were. The patient and her husband indicated they were

aware of the potential interaction, but she had "forgotten it." Apparently, an adverse interaction pop-up did not occur from the computer when her dismissal medications were prescribed.

Dr. Wise seemed as concerned with excusing Dr. Thueban's negligence as he'd been with diagnosing me. The physician assistant who'd prescribed the Lamisil/terbinafine had told me about the contraindication, but I *had* forgotten the conversation! I'd forgotten almost everything that had happened between February and July of 2014!

And I'd never thought Thueban's *intent* was to cause harm. But that didn't matter. This part of the record was written for a judge or a jury, not for me or any subsequent treating physicians.

I'd run into the thin white coat line. Among police, there's an unwritten code of conduct called the thin blue line. It dictates that cops cover for one another's behavior, right or wrong. The same thing was clearly in effect among physicians.

I spun my wedding ring as I sat in Dr. Iyilik's office. "Dr. W-W-Wise says I have tardive dyskinesia. He thinks the high do-dose of amitriptyline that Thueban gave me pushed my brain over the edge, especially s-since it was pr-pre-scribed with the te-ter-binafine. He said my brain go-go-got set up by meep, long ter-term psych drug use, but the a-ami-amitriptyline pushed me over the edge."

"That makes sense," Dr. Iyilik replied. I glanced up and saw he was nodding slowly. He seemed sad. "I'm sorry I didn't see blah contraindication when I continued to prescribe the amitriptyline. I rely on the pharmacy to catch blah things. I won't blah on them anymore. Let's reduce blah amitriptyline dose right away. We'll get you off as soon as possible."

When he'd originally prescribed the low dose of twenty-five milligrams of amitriptyline, I hadn't been taking terbinafine. His only error had been in continuing to prescribe it once the terbinafine had been added in.

I met with Grace the next day. "Do you think I have borderline personality disorder?" I asked.

"I don't really believe in labels. Involving labels blah usually a less effective approach than treating the patient as an individual. You need them blah insurance but—no, if a label has to be used, that's not right. You definitely don't have borderline personality disorder."

"You were given that diagnosis in an institution. Institutions like labels. Male doctors especially love blah use labels to explain away the inconvenience of intelligent female patients. That's what that was about. I'm sure the doctor blah uncomfortable with you wanting to have a say in your treatment. You didn't want to go to groups. I've been seeing you for months blah I would've recommended you avoid the triggers of interacting with addicts in the groups, which is what you did.

"But he didn't ask *why* you avoided groups," she continued. "He didn't think blah needed to ask. He thought he knew. Because he's the *doctor*. You didn't do everything you were told to do. That's a threat to the way of blah institution. A label of borderline personality disorder alleviates that threat.

"I'll tell you a story," she went on. "When I was young, I saw something happen in a hospital. There was a woman patient there with a PhD in chemistry. When the doctors wanted to give her a drug, she asked for more information about it. She wanted to know what she was being told to take. The doctors were very irritated that she had the nerve to question their order. I heard two young male doctors, resident doctors, younger than her, talking about what a pain in the ass she was, how she thought she knew things."

I listened hard. The longer I sat and talked with someone and assimilated the nuances of their voice, the easier it was to understand them.

"Wow," I said. "A PhD in chemistry is prob-prob-probably a better degree with which to understand the f-f-foundations of pharmacology than an MD—"

"Right," Grace said. "But that didn't matter. They were the *doctors. They tell you. You* don't question. And she was a female. And she was confident. She asserted herself in the face of their authority.

The same thing happened when you went to the ER. The doctor said *conversion disorder* because institutions like to blame the victim. I thought it might've been the ECT. I've seen lots of my patients have ECT and lose functioning. I saw one of my older patients die shortly after starting ECT—but I'm not a neurologist." Her brows had pushed together, and her eyes looked damp.

What Grace said made sense. The rest of our society was like that, biased and easily influenced by symbols of power. Symbols of power included education, professional status, and, of course, masculinity. Why would medical culture be immune to these influences? Doctors are humans who live within the same social order as me—an order that rewards dominance and arrogance. They were just playing by the rules. They were just trying to win a losing game.

*How'd you feel when you started to uncover the dynamics that underlie health care culture, like the thin white coat line and the politics behind a borderline personality disorder diagnosis?*

How'd I feel? Relieved. I mean, I'd had a sense the whole time, and by the whole time I mean that since I'd first walked into a therapist's office—that something dirty was going on. It felt just like it'd felt when I was young and I had realized Mom was lying about me being white. Here I was being told by doctors and therapists to accept things that were contrary to my lived experience.

I'd spent years doing everything I was told to do by therapists and psychiatrists, and I just kept getting sicker. Then my brain got fucked, and I got treated like that was my fault. It was obvious to me that something was very wrong with the advice I was getting, but I kept second-guessing myself.

I mean, there's confidence, which is great, and I finally had some. But then there's conventional thought, and that tells you to trust people who are more educated than you in specific areas. It tells you those people will give you good, well-researched advice. My core feeling was self-assurance. I was learning to trust myself even more, and to accept that when something looks dirty, it probably is.

"The dogs are angry," I said as I inched away from our husky. The sound of her tongue against her paw was like the grinding of a power sander. The black rings of fur circling her eyes looked menacing.

"No, they're not, honey," Andrew said. "No one's angry. The dogs love you."

I spun and hit the wall as I tried to run from the room where the ferocious canines reclined on the floor. The Lupron had stopped the depression, but in its place were constant panic and a state of paranoia that came on every evening.

Dr. Iyilik was out of the country. I called Dr. Boatbill's office.

"Um, uh, hi, meep. This is Twilah Hiari. I'm calling for an um appointmeep with Dr. Boatbill."

"Oh, Twilah. Hello, please blah-blah moment," she said.

After a moment, she returned to the line. "Dr. Boatbill won't see blah anymore because of the lapse in your treatment."

I sorted through her words, pressed end, sat back, and closed my eyes.

I got a letter in the mail dated September 10, 2014.

*Dear Twilah:*

*Good care requires good follow-up and adherence to medical recommendations.*

*You were last seen in this office on March 25, 2014. On this date, you were advised and scheduled to follow up with me in three weeks. Your appointment was made for April 22, 2014. This appointment was canceled when your husband called and stated that you were being admitted to Local Hospital and that you were going to be administered ECT.*

*The next communication we received was a call stating that you had been advised to increase your antidepressant by your treating ECT physician. I agreed to the increase since you were being treated by that doctor, and it was ultimately his decision what would be best for you at that time.*

*The increase in your antidepressant was the last communication from you or from your treating physician before you called urgently on September 9, 2014, stating you were experiencing an adverse reaction to medications that you were administered by Local Hospital. This situation would not be appropriate for me to address, given the fact that I have not been kept up to date on your medications, doses, or treatment schedules. You were informed by my staff that you needed to contact your current treating physician.*

*The typical course of ECT is two to three weeks. At the end of the treatment, our office should have been provided with medical records and an appointment should have been made in my office for a follow-up appointment. Even during maintenance ECT, you should have been seeing me regularly. Since I received no prescription refill requests, no medical records, no phone calls, and no scheduled appointments from you, it was my understanding that you were choosing not to continue seeing me and that you were being seen by another physician who was handling your care.*

*As you were told by my staff when you called, if you are unhappy with your treatment by Local Hospital, or by your treating physician, you should contact your insurance company or local mental health care center to find a new physician.*

*Sincerely,*
*Feather Boatbill M.D.*

**I see Boatbill's point about how she couldn't address an adverse reaction caused by another prescriber.**

Well, yeah, I do too. But the larger case she's trying to make is bullshit. I'd had far longer lapses in treatment with her, and she'd never even hinted it was a problem. For her to say ECT lasts two to three weeks and that I should've contacted her and done this, that, and the other is ludicrous. First of all, my ECT lasted from April 23 to June 16. And she'd given me zero direction on what to do afterward. She expected me to abide by guidelines she'd never communicated.

I explained the situation with Dr. Boatbill to Grace. "That's ridiculous," Grace agreed. "But some of these psychiatrists are like a lot of these therapists. They want simple and easy. What you're dealing with is more complex, and they don't want to put time and effort into helping complex patients."

"But it's what they get paid to do!" I shook my head and let out a puff of disbelief.

"Of course it is. But some clinicians don't want to do the hard work. They want a quick fix—a few visits and you're on-your-way-type thing. It's very unfortunate."

"Yeah, yeah it is. Well, Boatbill and her patient abandonment aren't my problem anymore. I'll see what the State Board of Healing Arts thinks about it." I shrugged.

"Good!" chimed Grace. "Accountability is critical." She continued, "So, are you up for talking more about your childhood today?"

"Sure, why not?" I nodded. I sat back and rested my hands on my knees. I shifted my focus to my breath to prepare myself for the discussion.

*Bang!* The noise came from the street. I jumped up and immediately began to feel disoriented. I looked out the window. A trash truck had dropped a bin from its mechanical claw. The sound of the truck's engine grew louder as it rolled down the street in our direction.

"Oh-oh," I said. My thoughts were becoming scrambled.

Grace got up and opened a closet door. She reached in and retrieved a small white box. She spoke as she plugged it into an outlet. She pushed a switch on the box and a soft staticky sound filled the room.

"Is that better?" she asked.

"Y-y-yes." While it was harder to hear her, it was easier to think. It would have to do.

"I don't like those trash trucks either," she said as she returned to her seat. "I saw one blah those trash men yell at my elderly neighbor about where he'd set his trash can along the curb. It was horrible.

Blah never seen a human being berate another human being like this. The driver was red in blah face, screaming at my elderly neighbor like he was a-a-a I don't know what. It blah unbelievable. I'd never seen blah human being behave that way."

"Lucky y-y-ou," I said with a small laugh. She'd somehow lived to midlife without ever having encountered a raging maniac. Raging maniacs had been ubiquitous in my youth. I wondered how she could be a therapist if her life had been so sheltered.

"When you had the third terrible stepfather, what was his name, the one who abused the animals—why didn't you tell anyone?" She was redirecting the conversation.

"I d-d-did tell people. I called the p-p-police on Java Man, er, George for beating the dogs and stuff, and the dispatcher laughed at me. A few weeks after that, my mom took me to Rainbow Mental Health. I think it was Rainbow. It was a therapy place down by KU Med. I know she was hoping to get rid of me. My mom took m-m-me to Rainbow and made this big display of how messed up I was, how I didn't get along with my stepfather. *Locking horns*, she called it. She said I was always locking horns with Java Man and that I was this bad, crazy kid. Locking horns. What does that even mean? I don't have any freaking horns!" I took a breath and waited for my rage to dissipate.

"They as-s-signed me a therapist. She must have been in her early twenties. S-s-skinny white girl. This therapist asked me why I wasn't getting along with my family. I tried to explain, 'Well, my stepfather's a raging madman.' I hoped she'd report it to the state. I hoped I'd get put in foster care or a group home like Glen, but that's not what happened."

"What happened?" Grace asked.

"S-s-so I tried to tell her what a madman George was, and this girl, this therapist, had interrupted me and started in on a lecture about the importance of compromise—how even if I didn't agree with how George and my mom lived, I needed to stop being uncooperative and g-go with the flow. I told her about how he was always high on drugs and raging. And she was like, 'W-w-well drugs aren't as bad as they preach in school.' She didn't want to talk about it anymore when I told her I didn't want to compromise.

"She changed the subject and asked if I had a boyfriend. I said, 'Yeah, I'm dating this guy.' She was like, 'Oh cool, tell me about him.' I said, 'Well, his name's Johnny Lee and he's thirty-six and he's really smart.'"

Grace's mouth opened. "You were just sixteen, right? What did she say when you told her you had a thirty-six-year-old boyfriend?"

"She said, 'Johnny Lee? Is he black? That sounds like a black name.' I said, 'No, he's white. He's in a band.' That really perked her up. She got excited and spent the next twenty minutes telling me about how she had a black boyfriend who was in a reggae band, and how he was amazingly awesome."

"Are you serious?" Grace's eyes widened.

"Yeah, I'm s-s-serious!"

"My God. I'm so sorry." Grace's lips turned down at the corners.

"Before that, my mom had made me go inpatient at Providence when I was thirteen. That's when my mom and Burt got divorced and my life went to hell."

"Did you explain the problems with your family to the staff at Providence?"

"No, no, I didn't. I didn't t-talk to them at all. I never spoke. They gave me dr-dr-drugs and forced me to take them. Finally, I spoke to ask the nurse if I could use the phone. I called Burt, and he came and got me released."

"Did the doctors there say you were depressed?"

"N-n-no, that's the funny thing. I remember for a long t-t-time afterward my mom had run around telling everyone I was sizzle frantic. I finally figured out she was saying schizophrenic. Idiots told her I had schizophrenia. I guess they said that because I stayed in my room and didn't talk to anybody. I didn't hear voices or hallucinate or anything. Schizophrenia! Idiots!" I shook my head and stared at my lap.

I glanced up when I heard Grace's voice. She was looking at me with her soft eyes. "How do you feel talking about all this?"

"Okay, really. I think it's good to get it off my chest." My heart rate was up; I could feel it. The sensation reminded me to bring my attention back to the rise and fall of my abdomen.

"Good, good. I think we're getting somewhere. I'll see you next week," said Grace.

# CHAPTER NINETEEN

THE TWANGY VOICE of a country singer boomed overhead. I put in my earbuds and tried to mask the sound with a white noise app, but I felt the inevitable acoustically induced confusion descend.

In the exam room, Soa, the gastroenterology physician assistant, positioned herself on a stool across from me. Even with a computer monitor in front of her, her large head loomed.

"Another specimen came back positive for C. diff?" Soa asked.

"Y-y-yes, it's b-back agaaaiiin," I replied.

"Your speech is slurred!" She whipped her enormous head around the side of the monitor and stared at me with narrowed eyes.

"I knowww," I replied. I'd been happy that I'd been able to speak at all that day, as the disconnect between my brain and my mouth was now so enormous.

"Why is your speech slurred?" she demanded. Her big head swung toward me, and her shoulders hunched up. I could tell she was angry at me, but I didn't understand why.

"Um, I saw this n-n-neurologist, Dr. Wise, and he said it's tardive dys-dyskinesia."

"Who's that?" she spat. Before I could answer, she was speaking again. "Did they give you anything for it?"

"Nooo—he said to wait and it will p-p-probableee goo away—"

"Really? I don't know about *that*!" Her words shot out hard and fast.

She crammed the rest of the appointment into less than five minutes. She kept peeking her gigantic head around the monitor and looking at me like I was some sort of revolting and dangerous creature. She hated me. Hated that I was there. Hated that she had to interact with me.

"Um. My mom has geee-eyyye problems too. She had so-so-some tests done heeere. Maybe I haaaave whatever she has?" In 2013, in an effort to establish a relationship with my mother, Andrew and I had taken her to see Dr. Vite for her distended abdomen and other ongoing medical issues.

Soa stared hard at me for a moment, then started typing. "What is your mother's name?"

"Uhhhh." I paused. "Deb, Deb, uh, Debbie, uh, Davenport?" I tried to remember which last name she currently had.

"How do you spell that?" Soa asked. "Debb-Y? Debb-IE? How?"

"I don't know," I answered after a long pause. I couldn't remember.

Soa stopped typing. Her head stretched around the monitor again, and she aimed another stony stare at me. I diverted my eyes to my lap.

"You don't know how to spell *your own mother's name*?"

I felt tears forming. I couldn't spell anything anymore. I couldn't write anymore.

"Well, I can't look your mother's condition up if you can't even spell her name. I've done all I can do with you. You need to see an infectious disease specialist. Dr. Blah-blah-blah-blah, you need to see him. The office will give you a call. Check out up front," she said before storming from the room.

I couldn't even begin to understand the name she'd said. It had several syllables and wasn't from any language with which I was familiar.

I wondered what I'd done to make Soa angry. *Does she think I'm drunk or on drugs because of my speech? Should I be worried about what Dr. Wise told me? Was Dr. Wise wrong?* Dr. Wise hadn't been very nice himself. Even though Soa was evil, that didn't mean she was wrong. Even assholes are right about things sometimes. Soa was an almost-doctor. *What's really happening to me?*

I went home and looked up neurologists. Dr. Vite sent a referral to a new one, and I was scheduled for his first available appointment, which was four months away.

No one from Soa's office called about a referral to the infectious disease specialist. I no longer used the phone because I could neither speak nor hear well. My efforts to listen and speak left me exhausted and confused. After Andrew left several messages with Soa's staff, someone finally called back and told him the time, date, and location of my appointment.

The infectious disease specialist's office was the sole occupant of a tiny strip mall in my hometown. The carpet in the waiting area was stained. The air smelled of nicotine and sweat. Hand-printed signs hung on the walls: LEAVE FOOD AND DRINK OUTSIDE.

A gum-popping woman in cartoon print scrubs called me back to an exam room. She waved for Andrew and me to take seats in hard plastic chairs.

The doctor walked in with a resident physician in tow. *Dr. Infectious*, I thought as the senior doctor introduced himself. I couldn't understand his name. His shirt was wrinkled, and his tie clung at an angle across it, glued there by static electricity. He leaned against the counter, shoulders stooped. He looked bored to the point of frustration.

The resident doctor looked young enough to be in high school. His wavy ginger hair was slightly greasy and uncombed. He shadowed the postures of the senior doctor, propping himself against the counter and rounding his shoulders. He squinted and lifted his chin as Dr. Infectious spoke. These two surly men looked like they belonged in a pool hall, not a doctor's office.

"You have C. diff?" Dr. Infectious asked. "You try vancomycin?"

"Yes, and Dificid too. She's allergic to Flagyl. She's had several courses of each. The C. diff has come and gone multiple times. It's refractory to antibiotic treatment," Andrew explained. Even though my speech had started to improve again, I'd given up speaking in these situations. Doctors were more receptive to Andrew anyway.

"Then it's time for a transplant," Dr. Infectious said. "We take bacteria from healthy feces and put it in your gut. It has the highest cure rate for C. diff, better than all antibiotics." He pushed himself away from the counter and stood in front of me, arms crossed against his chest. It felt like he disapproved of my very existence. After he turned and left the room, Andrew and I hurried out.

The transplant was considered experimental, so it wasn't covered by insurance. We pinched pennies, and in September 2014, I had a fecal transplant via a bacteria pill. After the transplant, the C. diff I'd been battling for months was cured.

*Why hadn't anyone ordered a transplant sooner? Why'd you have to suffer for so long?*

Good question.

# CHAPTER TWENTY

THE MOUNTAINS ROSE up in the distance, and the air felt clear and cool. I leaned against my hiking poles and breathed in the sharp scent of evergreens. The fingers of my right hand worked my mala. I softly chanted a mantra for healing and purification.

I was back in Colorado. A couple Andrew knew had gifted us their timeshare for a week. I gazed beyond the evergreens to the pulsing yellows and oranges of the aspens in the valley below. Gratitude filled my heart. My cyclical depression was gone, and an amazingly generous pair of human beings had materialized and given us a vacation.

"You ready, honey?" Andrew's voice brought me back. I'd paused because each step I took was now paired with what felt like a shock from my heel to my jaw. I told myself to breathe, to ignore the pain and focus on the scenery.

"Yeah, yeah, I'm ready," I said as I wrapped my mala around my left wrist. "Can we head back down?"

"Sure. Let's go back to town and get something to eat," Andrew agreed.

My steps had become short and mincing. Tears rose up in response to the pain shooting through my feet and legs. I put all the weight I could on my hiking poles. Back at the hotel, I soaked in the hot tub and roasted in the sauna.

Each hike brought the same pain, which I tried to ignore. I didn't want my body to ruin our trip. When we were alone, high up in the mountains, away from the city and its sounds, my speech became clearer and my anxiety less intense.

A day into our stay, the skin on my calves broke out in small, itchy red blisters. I searched the hotel room for bugs but didn't see any. I'd worn insect repellent during our hikes and hadn't been bitten by anything. I asked the housekeeping staff to rewash our bedding in water only, without detergent or fabric softener. When the sheets were returned to the bed, the blisters on my legs disappeared.

A woman I knew from my teens had been texting me nonstop since she'd learned I was going to Colorado. She told me I needed to try the marijuana, which was legal in the state. "It'll cure anything," she'd gushed. Weed had never been my thing, but in the context of the excruciating pain in my bones, I thought it was worth a try.

In a store outside Leadville, I picked out an edible that was supposed to have cannabidiol (CBD), the component that's used to treat pain and inflammation, without tetrahydrocannabinol (THC), the component that's supposed to make you feel high.

After a long bath, I'd broken off a piece of the bar the size of my fingertip, half of the recommended starting dose. Despite the quiet in the room, anxiety descended. I'd focused on my breath and drifted into sleep. I awoke to a crashing sound. Someone had broken in! I struggled to open my eyes. A gigantic man in a cowboy hat swaggered toward me.

"You got a problem with me?" he roared. His head was an enormous, seven-pointed leaf. His lips were green and seeded.

*Oh my god. Oh my GOD! This is a dream. Take control. Take control!*

"Yeah, I've got a problem with you!" I shouted back. "Get out of my body!"

The CBD cowboy disappeared in a puff of smoke. I could feel the blood pumping through my veins, pulsing into my ears and eyes. I turned my focus to my breath, visualized the Buddha, and lapsed into more peaceful dreams.

❧

*Had you realized by then that your body doesn't process drugs like other people's bodies?*

Uh, yeah. I mean, Andrew noticed before I did. It was a mental thing for me. I'd grown up with Mom constantly complaining about her health problems and how she was so different from other people physiologically. She'd literally gone around saying, "Doctors can't figure out what's wrong with me. It's because I'm an alien!"

I didn't want to be like that. I didn't want to be like her in any way. So, I was kinda in denial about this pattern of side effects until Andrew was like, "Damn, you have the worst reactions to every drug. It's crazy!" And I had to accept that yeah, I'm pretty prone to adverse reactions.

*Does your mom actually have any rare illnesses?*

I never thought she did, because of her lies and her hyperbole. But now I wonder. She had something happen to her brain. She calls it, "When my head blew up." She describes this sudden onset of migraines, vision problems, and bilateral tinnitus, all of which fluctuated with barometric pressure. She also said her menopause was a nightmare that made her act crazy. Then she's had this grossly distended abdomen for the last twenty or so years, and a colonoscopy and ultrasound don't show anything amiss. I mean, this isn't make believe. She's seventy-three years old and has this rock-hard gut that makes her look nine months pregnant.

She's generally unhealthy. She's diabetic. She's had skin cancer, breast cancer, cervical cancer, two strokes. She's had a ton of problems. Her lifestyle's terrible. She eats nothing but processed foods. She's smoked since she was a teenager. She never exercises. You'd expect poor health, right? But some of the symptoms that she hasn't gotten diagnoses for are really weird.

～

While we were in Colorado, Andrew had called Sara, Dr. Fahrig's nurse, and told her about the crippling pain I'd had during our hikes.

Sara wrapped the blood pressure cuff around my arm. "I see y'all are back home. Are you feeling any better? I passed your message on to Dr. Fahrig. I'm sorry you had all that pain during y'alls vacation. I'd say it's about time y'all caught a break."

"Oh, thank you. It's not your fault. I'm feeling better now, thank goodness. I just don't understand what's going on," I said.

"Well, y'all have been dealing with a lot. I hope Dr. Fahrig can help y'all get this figured out. She'll be here in a few minutes. You two take care," she said as she noted my metrics in the chart.

"Thank you. You too," I offered. I wondered why more nurses weren't nice like Sara.

When Dr. Fahrig came in, I gave her an update. "My mood's great. The depression's gone. I just have anxiety and confusion. My speech isn't perfect, but it's better a lot of the time. But man, the pain I had when we were hiking in Colorado was unbelievable!"

"The pain you describe is call arthralgia. It can be a side effect of Lupron," she said.

"Well, it was horrible, and I still get it when we try to walk in the park. I don't think I can do the Lupron anymore."

"Okay. You've had three doses. The improvement in your mood since you started it proves your depression was hormone related. We'll stop the injections. You'll have a big rebound of hormones though, and your depression will probably come back. Follow up with me in a few weeks."

The arthralgia became less pronounced as the Lupron left my body, but back in the city, away from the peace of the mountains, everything was still so loud.

～

"Would you please refund this fee?" I asked. We'd dealt with the banker, Megan, on several occasions. Each time we'd worked with her, she'd cheerfully screwed up each of our transactions.

"The banking agreement says it's only supposed to be charged on accounts that don't have direct deposit, and my husband's check gets directly deposited."

"No, I can't," Megan said with a small smile. "Fees are nonrefundable."

As soon as I'd deciphered her words, I'd felt the rage. "Refund this fucking fee! Now!" I slammed my purse down and lunged across the desk at her.

Megan leapt from her chair and stumbled against the desk behind her.

"You need to leave! Leave now, or I'm going to call the police! You are banned from ever coming into this branch again!" she shouted in a trembling voice.

"You need to give me my fucking money!" I shouted back.

Andrew had grabbed my elbow and was pulling me from the building.

"Come on, come on," he begged. "This isn't worth it. We don't have money for bail."

That bitch had just put me over the top. But my rage wasn't right. It just wasn't right. Everyone makes mistakes. *What was wrong with me?*

In the car, I squeezed my eyelids shut. I felt my brain swelling and pushing against my skull. Behind our car, a man poured glass from a cardboard box into a recycling bin. The sound shot like an ice pick through my ears.

"Oh my God, oh my God, oh my God! I'm gonna die! This is killing me!" I shrieked as I slapped my hands over my ears. Tears streamed as pain ripped across my brain.

⁕

"My pain in my body's better. But I have this rage and fear. The level of my anger is literally frightening to me," I reported to Dr. Fahrig at my next appointment.

"The anger you describe is also a side effect of the Lupron. Now, you might understand those older women we all have in our families, the ones that turn so angry that it makes you wonder what's gone wrong with sweet old grandma. Disruption of your hormones can result in extreme anger," assured Dr. Fahrig with a gentle smile.

"Well, it's horrible," I said. I didn't have a grandma to relate her comment to, but I'd seen plenty of angry old women.

"We'll keep an eye on this. I'll see you again in a few weeks," Dr. Fahrig said.

―

"How've you been? Have there been any changes to your symptoms?" Dr. Wise asked.

"Okay. My mouth and jaw movements have been improving, but I have this horrible anxiety. I saw a different psychiatrist last week—that was the end of October, right? Anyway, she prescribed Fetzima for it. As soon as I started the Fetzima, the mouth movements came back. When that happened, I stopped taking it. But the anxiety and panic were still there, so Dr. Vite prescribed Zoloft. The Zoloft brought back the movements, and I started to feel confused again. I'm still confused a lot of the time. And my short-term memory's still awful." I shrugged as I wrapped up my explanation.

"Your speech is much clearer; I think that's a positive. I'm not familiar with Fetzima. It must be new. I still think if you get to a point where you're able to avoid all psychoactive drugs and antiemetics, your movement problems may resolve on their own," he repeated the advice he'd offered before.

I wasn't sure I could trust him. Soa had planted a seed of doubt in my mind about his competence. But I did my best to follow his directions.

Days later, I took my final dose of amitriptyline. My speech cleared up even more, and my mouth and jaw movements calmed down a lot. Instead of stuttering and slurring my words, I had long pauses between words and sentences. And I didn't say *meep* or *bay* much anymore.

But as the Lupron left my system, the depression came rushing back. And as Fahrig had predicted, it was more intense than ever. I felt like someone had thrown an executioner's hood over my head and was pushing a blade against my neck. I wanted to force the blade into my artery.

I explained my dilemma to Dr. Fahrig. "Since your mood is at such a dangerous low again, and you can't tolerate Lupron, we can consider a hysterectomy and oophorectomy," she said.

"Yes. Yes, please," I said after a pause. I'd struggled to visualize the letters that spelled *oophorectomy* in my mind, but once I saw them, the word glowed golden in my head. "Can we do it before the end of the year? My deductible's met, and I won't be able to afford it come January when I have a new deductible."

"I'll talk to the surgeon and see. I'll certainly do my best to make that happen. Sara will call you by next week."

Sara called a few days later. I listened through my earbuds. "We can schedule you on Christmas Eve. Nobody else wants surgery then, so the calendar's wide open."

"Yes, yes, I'll take it. Just tell me when to be there."

Later, when I saw Grace, I gushed, "I'm going to have a hysterectomy. It's gonna cure the PMDD!"

"How do you feel about that?" she asked.

"Great," I said. "I'm going to be cured!"

"Are you worried about it?" she continued.

"No, I'm not worried. The surgeon has a great reputation, and it's a low-risk procedure as far as major surgery goes—"

"Yes, but how do you *feel* about it?"

"Excited?" I offered. I thought I'd just told her how I felt about it.

Grace regarded me. "You don't have any kids," she said.

"No."

"Does that bother you, that you'll never have kids?"

"No. I really don't like kids. I only wanted a kid briefly when my hormones were out of control."

Grace continued to stare at me. I thought maybe I knew what she was getting at. I'd seen women launch into frenzies when they'd been told they needed a hysterectomy for one reason or another. I'd heard laments of "lost womanhood" and "stolen femininity." And I thought it was bullshit. I thought it was absolute crap. How could they identify so deeply with their ovaries and uteruses? You didn't hear about people losing their minds over appendectomy surgery. Maybe Grace expected me to be languishing in that foolishness.

"Well, it's clear to me that the worst of your depression was related to your hormones. I saw that when you started the Lupron. But there's something else I see. You never have any fun. You need to do something *fun*!"

I felt my brows come together.

"I have fun," I offered. "I have fun quilting and walking my dogs—and walking in the park with my husband, and meditating, and reading, and writing."

"No, I mean *fun*. I mean, you need to go to a *movie* or something. Go out somewhere!" She launched into a description of a movie her friend had seen and loved. I couldn't quite follow what she was saying—something about a funny movie about family problems. After several minutes, she stopped speaking.

"I hate movies," I said.

"You. Hate. Movies." She made it sound like I'd said *I kick puppies*.

"Yeah, I hate movies. I always have. I've only gone to them when other people invited me so that I seemed polite. I actually had some friends in my twenties who were always having movie nights. I watched movies with them every weekend, but I always zoned out. Movies don't make any sense to me. I've never understood why people like them."

Grace was still gazing at me. "Okay then. Good luck with your surgery. I'll see you in the new year."

# CHAPTER TWENTY-ONE

"BLAH, THIS IS blah. We only blah opening blah Christmas Eve," the woman said.

"Yeah, um, hi. I c-can do surgery Christmas Eve, but can I not have a roommate p-p-lease? I can't handle s-sounds like TV and pe-pe-people talking and stuff."

"You want a private room? Your insurance might not cover it," she replied. "Blah big out of pocket charge. Blah-blah."

"What?"

She repeated her statement about insurance and charges. As broke as we were, I didn't care. I'd risk years of debt to avoid hearing people chatting and the sounds of a television.

"Well, if you think you must have a private room, I'll mention it. It's not really in my control. That's up to the floor nurse." Her words had become clipped. Several whats and huhs later, I finally understood what she was saying.

"How do I contact the floor nurse?" I asked.

"You can't until you're in the hospital."

I shook my head and ended the call. I removed my earbuds, sat back, and closed my eyes. I'd never liked the phone, but now the effort of listening and speaking left me so drained, I had to follow each call with a nap.

※

"I'm so glad this is finally going to be over," Andrew said as he started the car.

"Me too," I replied. Christmas Eve had arrived. My gift would be freedom from PMDD.

At the hospital, a nurse inserted an IV into a vein and I drifted off to sleep. I woke up in another room.

"How are you feeling?"

I looked over at my husband, who was sitting in a chair to my right.

I pressed my head into the pillow, listened to my breath, and considered his question.

"I feel a calmness I haven't felt in years."

He leaned over and kissed my forehead. His eyes were moist.

A young nurse strode into the room.

"Oh, you're awake!" she proclaimed. "You want this TV on?"

"No!" my husband and I shouted in unison.

Her head jerked back a bit.

"Okay then," she drawled. "Oh yeah, you're the need-a-private-room-cuz-she-hates-noise lady."

Her eyes were slit as she regarded me.

"Huh?" I said. What she'd said finally sunk in. I guessed word had gotten around about my need for quiet without me having to ask for a floor nurse.

She ran her fingers through her hair with her gloved hand, then started manipulating my IV where it entered my arm. I was horrified at the unhygienic act, but my speech wouldn't come. Andrew had left to use the restroom.

"Blah-blah Christmas—blah-blah—IKEA—blah-blah-blah—my kids—blah-blah—I delivered my son here blah-blah last year," spilled from her mouth. The pace of her speech was impossible to follow. I felt my brain slowing and confusion setting in. I closed my eyes and fell back asleep.

The next day, a different nurse checked on me. She told me I could go home that afternoon. She handed me a blue package full of disposable wipes. "You can use these to clean yourself up."

I hobbled to the bathroom and wiped the crusted blood from my abdomen and thighs. Within minutes, the area that I'd touched with the wipes was swollen and oozing. Like flaming red hills, hives had arisen across the landscape of my lower body.

"Another reaction. My God, you can't tolerate anything!" said Andrew. He shook his head and wore a faint expression of disbelief. "That's just raw. You're gonna need a prescription for that."

The physician assistant who saw me afterward at Suburban Clinic was intrigued. "So, after you cleaned yourself with the wipes, you broke out in these hives and started having urinary frequency and urgency? Interesting. You have quite the history of reactions, don't you?" she said as she scrolled through my records.

"Hives from ibuprofen, rashes from one, two, three, four, *five* different medications. Visual disturbances with Flagyl—oh and you've been sick a lot this year too. Hives, bronchitis, an abscess, C. diff—oh C. diff, I'm so sorry. I'm going to have to do some looking to make sure I treat this properly."

"G-great, I appreciate your thoroughness," I said. I was willing to wait all day for her to research a safe treatment.

After a couple of minutes of reading, she turned back toward us. "I'm pretty sure we'll be okay with Depo-Medrol, but I do see a small contraindication with it and the estradiol patch you're on for hormone replacement. Because of that, I'd like to give you a lower dose of the Depo-Medrol, not the full dose, and supplement it with a steroid cream. How does that sound?"

"Um, sounds reasonable to me," I replied after I'd sorted through her words.

Another nurse injected the Depo-Medrol into a fleshy area near my hip. Within hours, my speech had become slurred and I had begun to stutter again. My confusion and strange mouth movement returned as well.

❦

Six days after my hysterectomy, I pushed myself out of bed and got into the shower. It was time for my appointment with the movement disorder specialist.

My phone rang as we drove to the appointment. "Hello?" I answered.

"Hi, this is Lacy with patient advocacy. You left me a message?"

"Yes, hi, t-t-thanks for calling me back. I was just calling to r-r-report an allergic reaction to some wipes I was given after my surgery. I thought you should know, so that you could consider warning p-p-patients of any potential issues." I noticed I was struggling with my speech again.

"Oh." Her chirpy voice now had a low tone. "We can't warn everybody about anything and everything. People react to all kinds of things—the sheets, the soap, whatever. That's not something that needs to be addressed. Is that all you wanted?"

I paused to process what she'd said. "I guess so." I pressed end.

"Who was that?" asked Andrew.

"The p-p-patient advocate I called to t-t-tell about the allergic reaction to the w-w-wipes. She b-b-b-basically doesn't give a shit." My head felt muddled from the effort of engaging in the call.

"I'm not surprised," said Andrew. "Your raw, oozing stomach and legs and your need to go to your primary care provider's office for a steroid injection are obviously a gigantic waste of her precious time."

"Obviously," I concurred.

We parked, and I walked as quickly as I could through the frosty air and into the lobby. I put in my earbuds and surveyed the waiting area. I appeared to be the only patient under the age of sixty-five in the room. A nurse who looked old enough to be in the waiting room herself called us back. She asked for the paperwork I'd been sent. I handed her the packet Andrew had helped me complete, which included a report of no findings from the brain MRI Dr. Wise had ordered. I also offered her a sheet I'd created that outlined all of my symptoms, their times of onset, and the medication exposures that had preceded my symptoms. But she waved it away.

"I only want what they sent you in the mail," she said. "So, tell me why you're here."

It was hard to speak again since the Depo-Medrol injection had prompted the return of the worst of my cognitive and movement problems. Andrew did most of the explaining of what had transpired. I wondered why she couldn't just read the sheet I'd offered her that had the full synopsis.

"Twilah's had PMDD for several years. It kept getting misdiagnosed as major depressive disorder. She resorted to ECT, because the PMDD made her suicidal," Andrew offered.

"PM what?" asked the nurse.

Andrew launched into a detailed tutorial on PMDD. He'd become quite an expert on the subject.

"Okay," said the nurse, "what else?"

"When she was in the hospital for ECT, she contracted C. diff, which was refractory to antibiotic treatment. She had that on and off from May through September of this year. It was cured by a fecal transplant," he explained.

"Oh, oh my," said the nurse. "Poor you!"

"That's not all," continued Andrew. "In July, she had a severe reaction to a Lupron injection. It affected her cognition, and she lost the ability to read and count. When she sought treatment for that, she was overdosed on amitriptyline by an incompetent psychiatrist. That's when this mouth movement and her other movement problems started. She also lost the ability to speak. She still can't speak all the time."

"That's a rough year," the nurse said.

"Yeah, it's kinda sucked," I offered.

"Dr. Crow will be in shortly," she said when she finished typing.

A few minutes later, a man in a white coat entered the room. I could smell his breath before I could see the pattern on his tie. He introduced himself, then asked me to stand and walk from one end of the room to the other.

With effort, I pushed myself up from the chair. I did my best to follow his instructions. His words came out fast and sharp. I struggled to understand them. I could tell from his pinched expression that he wasn't happy with my performance. He waved at me to have a seat again.

"It h-hurts," I tried to explain. "I j-just had a hysterectomy s-six days ago."

I lifted the bottom of my shirt to reveal the incisions.

"I don't need to see it!" he shouted.

I dropped the hem of my shirt and sat back. I wondered why he was angry. I'd only showed him because he didn't seem to understand why it hurt me to walk.

He squatted in front of me and barked out instructions: "Move your eyes here." "Move your hands here." I tried my best, but I couldn't keep up with his speech. I started to cry.

"Oh, you need to stop crying," Dr. Crow barked. "Do we need to reschedule because you have to cry?"

*Oh my God no*, I thought. I'd waited months for this appointment. I needed information!

"No," I said through my tears. "It's just that it hurts and I'm so c-c-confused."

Dr. Crow stepped back and positioned himself near the window. Light reflected off his forehead where he had no hair left to cover it.

"This is *not* tardive dyskinesia. This is a psychogenic movement disorder. You are not doing it on purpose. It isn't your fault. The treatment for it is dialectical behavioral therapy. If you do that, it will go away." He crossed his arms across his chest as he spoke.

It took me a moment to absorb what he'd said. I was still staring at his mouth when I opened mine to respond. "So, wh-what accounts for the difference between y-y-your opinion and Dr. Wise's opinion?"

"I will not be a party to you accusing Dr. Wise of malpractice! Don't you think you can run out and get a lawyer now," he roared.

"Dr. Wise sent you to me because I'm an expert on movement disorders!"

But Dr. Wise hadn't sent me. I'd sent myself. And I hadn't meant anything about malpractice. I took several breaths and reached for clarity.

"Wh-wh-what? What I meant was—why did my movement symptoms start with the amitriptyline and come back when I took Zoloft, F-Fetzima, and Depo-Medrol? Dr. Wise said those medications caused it, but you seem to be saying s-s-something else."

"It's part of your conversion disorder," Dr. Crow said. "You need to stop this questioning me and focus on getting better."

"I'm just tr-tr-trying to understand," I pleaded through my tears. "I w-w-want to understand."

I pulled out the list and timeline I'd composed. "What about these other symptoms, not just my mouth movement and speech problems. What about my c-confusion and memory loss. My p-problems with r-reading—my inability to t-tolerate—"

"I've been doing this for years," Dr. Crow interrupted. "I see this three or four times *a week* in my practice. I know what it is. You need to accept it. You need to focus on fixing your emotional problems if you want to get better. Dr. Wise sent you to me for a reason. I am *the expert* on this! Any more questions?" he spat. He'd sat down at his computer, and the clacking of the keyboard echoed inside of my head.

The only question on the tip of my slightly protruding tongue was, "Are all neurologists fucking assholes?" But I turned my focus to my breath and swallowed the words. Dr. Crow stood up and left the room. We saw ourselves out.

We'd traveled several miles before I could speak again.

"That Bilbo Baggins h-h-hobbit-ass looking mother-f-f-fucker needs to crawl back in his hobbit hole. May the hair on his toes choke his—oh, this is wrong speech." I stopped. I had so much work to do to achieve anything that approximated compassion and loving kindness in these stressful situations.

Andrew laughed so hard he spat out his coffee. "Well, at least you still have a way with words," he said.

The next day, I plugged in my earbuds and called Dr. Crow's office. The person who answered sent me to his nurse's voicemail. I did my best to leave a message asking for a coherent explanation for why my symptoms always worsened with exposure to medications. I was pretty sure that with my ovaries gone, my depression would stay away. But what if it didn't? Dr. Wise had been insistent that I avoid all the drugs that had ever triggered my reactions. I needed to know for sure whether medications were safe or not.

The nurse called me back a few hours later. It was the same older woman who'd seemed so sympathetic when I'd checked in.

"I took your question about medications to Dr. Crow. He said he told you yesterday that you don't need medication for your disorder," she huffed. I paused as I sorted through her words.

"That wasn't my question. I'm sorry if that w-w-wasn't clear on the voicemail, but I wasn't asking for dr-dr-drugs. I was asking w-w-why I react so badly to drugs. Why does my sp-sp-speech worsen with exposure to medication?" I struggled to respond.

"Because it's part of your disorder!" she shrieked.

"*How* is it part of my disorder? I'm looking for an answer w-w-with content please," I replied with great difficulty. My ears hurt. My brain hurt.

"It just is!" she was still shrieking. "It's part of your diagnosis!"

"So, if s-s-someone wants to prescribe me antidepressants in the future th-th-then, can I take them?"

"Antidepressants won't help your condition!" she shouted.

*Are these people more cognitively disabled than me?* "Why am I encountering s-s-ooo much hostility from this office?" I countered.

"Because you won't listen! Because you won't accept your diagnosis! That's why!" she continued shouting in my ear. "Dr. Crow is the best. People come from all over to see him. All over! He's booked out for months because he's the most knowledgeable. You need to *accept your diagnosis!*"

"I don't c-c-care who comes from where to see him. That's

irrelevant. Why. Can't. I. G-g-get an answer with s-s-substance and content to m-m-my question?"

"Dr. Crow told you! Now I'm telling you! *That's your answer!*" she yelled.

I pressed end.

I logged onto Facebook to vent. I was greeted by a meme celebrating the sacrifices and heroism of nurses. I tapped out a misspelled and hostile response. I can't remember exactly what I wrote, but it was something to the effect of how respect should only be afforded to people who treat others with respect and how nurses often behaved disrespectfully. I came under swift attack from a pack of nurses and nurse worshippers.

A nurse practitioner private messaged me: *You just need to be more positive! Your negative attitude is your problem!* she chided. *I had a rough time a couple of years ago and I chose a positive attitude. Now I'm fine!*

I knew from Andrew that Nurse Quaff was an alcoholic who used an app on her phone to diagnose her patients. She hadn't chosen a positive attitude; she'd chosen to buy her hooch by the case instead of the bottle.

Criticizing nurses, I learned, had the equivalent social effect of erecting an effigy of Satan in a Baptist sanctuary. My criticism of nurses came close to wiping out my friend list.

In many ways, Facebook was all I had left. In the years since I'd become sick with PMDD, my few friends had moved away to the coasts or out of the country entirely. I could no longer have phone conversations, and people of my generation tend to prefer the phone to email or text. Because of these barriers, old friendships that I thought I'd be able to revive with my recovery from PMDD evaporated.

The few people I interacted with locally knew nothing of what was going on. They rambled on about their lives as I sat silently, smiling and nodding intermittently, unable to figure out how or when to interject. The few times I'd tried to speak, to ask for support for what I was going through, people had cut me off or talked over me, just like they'd always done.

The people I knew didn't have time for the struggles of others. Nobody gave the slightest shit about me until I blew a gasket and violated some social holy grail by criticizing the medical establishment in general, or God forbid, nurses in particular. Then they raced out of the woodwork with their condemnation and tone policing.

*Let's talk about this segment. Lots of my patients tell me that after they've gone through a major illness, they feel like they learn who their true friends are afterward. Do you feel that's what happened to you?*

That's not really what I meant. What I meant is I found where peoples' biases are. When I responded to the nurse worship meme, I had people who are otherwise sensible, but happen to have a friend or family member who's a nurse, lash out at me.

I mean, I got hit with pure hatred from people who stand up for other civil right issues—people who are dedicated advocates for equal rights when it comes to race or sexual orientation. But those same people refused to acknowledge the civil rights violation that is medical abuse.

But that's only the negative. I learned something good from this too. You know who stood by me, no questions asked? The few disabled people I knew, that's who. Because every last one of them has been treated like shit by a nurse or a doctor at some point, simply because they'd showed up to purchase medical treatment on the wrong damned day. They'd showed up when someone was in a bad mood, had a long shift, wanted to be at the Royals game, needed to go pick up their kids—whatever.

It's like anything. If you don't do something often, you're less likely to see all the facets of it. If you're disabled or chronically ill, and you have to go see doctors all the goddamned time, you're going to get treated like shit by nurses and doctors a lot more often than if you only go for a physical once a year.

I learned that if I needed someone to have my back, it would be someone with a disability or at least someone who'd dealt with a major health episode. That's where I'd find my allies.

# CHAPTER TWENTY-TWO

"THERE'S NO REASON to ever treat a patient like that," Grace declared after I told her about my appointment with Dr. Crow and my phone call with his nurse.

"Well, yeah. But what about th-this dialectical b-b-behavioral therapy thing he mentioned? Is there any merit to it?"

"I've been trained in dialectical behavioral therapy, and I'm qualified to employ it. I choose not to. As you know, I utilize cognitive behavioral therapy. DBT may be useful for a small number of patients with a very limited range of challenges. I don't see it as being appropriate in your case.

"Crow's office clearly has a sick culture. They had no respect for your need for information. I know you, and I know that's how you heal, by processing things intellectually. If they were so quick to treat you so badly just because you asked for an explanation, that tells me this isn't the first time that's happened. Substandard treatment of patients is something that's habitual and accepted there. Like any abuse from any source, you don't have to take the burden on yourself. It stems from *their* issues, and you must take care not to internalize it."

I listened carefully. I could see some of the words she spoke. What she said made sense.

"Well, it was h-h-hard for me to make the phone call, but I w-w-want information. I think I'm going to send them a letter."

"That is a very good idea," Grace replied. "Use your voice."

*1/1/2015*

*Dear Dr. Crow,*

*I believe it is clear that our interaction at my scheduled appointment on 12/30, as well as my subsequent communication with your nurse, went badly. I would like to offer my perspective on the events that transpired. Prior to becoming unable to work, I was employed by two highly regarded Fortune 500 companies. At those locations, you would often hear spoken a phrase that pertained to customer relations. The phrase was, "They don't care how much you know until they know how much you care." Yes, cheesy and corporate, but I recommend you meditate on the concept.*

*It was not my intention to ask questions that made you uncomfortable or suspicious of ulterior or devious motives. Every question I posed was for the purpose of gaining insight into my condition or the methodology involved in the diagnosis. When you left the exam room so abruptly, I was given no choice but to call and leave my remaining questions with your nurse. I cannot recount them verbatim, but I intended to ask something along the lines of: a) In the context of your diagnosis, what accounts for the correlation between my exposure to antidepressants and the worsening of my condition? b) Can I resume, if advised to do so by a psychiatrist, to take antidepressants for depression, should I again experience depression?*

*I acknowledge I may not have worded my questions so precisely in my voicemail and have already apologized to your nurse if that is what instigated any misunderstanding. You will see why I was quite disappointed when your nurse advised me that the answer to question (a) was something along the lines of: "That is an aspect or* component of your condition." Let me offer an analogy. I present to my GP with the flu. I ask, "Why am I coughing so much?" GP replies, "It is a symptom of the flu."

*Accurate but unsatisfying. Instills no confidence in the diagnosis or practitioner. Better answer from GP, "The flu virus affects the respiratory system in such a way that . . ." Do you see the difference? Your nurse was very confrontational when I expressed dissatisfaction with the answer I received to my first question. She treated my continued inquiry as me rejecting my diagnosis, when what I was doing was seeking information. She became quite openly hostile.*

*She then offered in answer to (a) that you had seen the same occur in other patients with identical diagnoses. Great, but again, significantly lacking in actual content or information. Then she responded to question (b) that there is no point in attempting to treat my condition with psychoactive drugs. Yes, how utterly well I understand that. My question was not regarding the use of such drugs to treat THIS condition, but to treat any depression I may experience in the future.*

*The conversation was a complete failure, and as I have demonstrated, it was not a failure because of any refusal to listen on my part. Again, if my questions were not so clearly worded on the voicemail, I apologize, but there was absolutely no need for the degree of animosity I encountered in my conversation with your nurse. I asked her directly why I was encountering so much hostility from this office.*

*She indicated it was because I didn't want to listen. She then regaled me with semiworshipful statements about your unquestionable capabilities as a physician. Well, let me explain what qualifies a doctor as a good doctor, from the perspective of many patients. The ability to communicate effectively with many people with many different diagnoses is one criteria of a good physician. Another quality is expression of empathy. Declarations from Dr. Kim Jong Crow and Associates don't really instill confidence in a patient. Such declarations don't meet either of the above criteria. But perhaps that doesn't matter much to you. I mean, who really* cares what a patient thinks if you've published this and that and contributed this and that to the body of medical knowledge. If your hubris is such that such a thought process is permissible, then the effort at communication is pointless.

From here, I would still like answers to questions (a) and (b) as restated above. I will consider the answers thoughtfully. However, as the poor communication to date from you and your nurse has failed to instill in me complete confidence in your diagnosis, I will seek another opinion. I will not advise you from whom. My point is even with your big Great Crow Show you failed to instill confidence in me of your abilities. Write me off as a little nobody at your own peril. That is not a threat in any way, it is simply a reminder that you quite possibly never know with whom you are dealing and it is always prudent to make sure all of your patients and your patient's questions are treated with dignity and respect.

Sincerely,
Twilah Hiari

After many edits and spellchecks, I dropped it in the mail. I didn't get a response, not until I sent a second letter threatening legal action. When Dr. Crow wrote back, he explained that the medical literature since the early 1900s reports that people with conversion disorder have unusual responses to medications.

It took me several months to get the records from the visit. When I read them, I realized it had been like Dr. Crow and I had been on different planets instead of in the same room.

> She is alert and oriented in all spheres. Language functions are normal as are cognitive functions. She had trouble maintaining eye contact and cried after I attempted to test upper body (arm) strength stating that she was still sore from her surgery. She then proceeded to pull up her shirt to show me the incision and stitches. After being informed of my diagnosis, she returned several times asking me as to

why Dr. Wise did not get the same diagnosis. I tried several times to redirect her, and then I emphatically reminded her that the only reason she was seeing me was for my opinion so that she could get better. Why the diagnoses were different was not important compared to what to do to help her get better.

---

**Where specifically, was Crow's report off base?**

Where was it *not* off base? I mean, my language function was absolutely not normal! Here I was with this stammer and these long pauses between words. But Dr. Crow had never met me before, so how did he know how fluent I had or hadn't been before I saw him? And the same was true of my cognition. I knew damn well it was seriously impaired.

Most of the time, I couldn't see the words I wanted to say. My entire life I'd been able to visualize words. I need to visualize words in order to speak. I think of it as my internal closed captioning system. Now mind you, I didn't know at the time that my internal closed captioning was anything unusual. I just knew it had been there my entire life and it wasn't there anymore.

Andrew had tried to emphasize to Dr. Crow how smart I'd been before and how he could see that my problem-solving skills and memory weren't even close to what they'd once been. But Dr. Crow wasn't hearing it. And the eye contact thing. Ha! Yeah, eye contact had never been easy, but at this point it'd become almost impossible. Like the head banging, it was another regression to how I'd behaved when I was a child.

And I'd never said anything about pain in my arm. What I'd been trying to do was explain that I was having trouble walking and performing any movement that involved the stabilizing muscles of my abdomen. But what stands out most in my memory is I'd had an incredibly hard time understanding Dr. Crow and how frustrating that had been. So yeah, I wouldn't be surprised if I'd answered some of his questions wrong and made him think I meant that my arm hurt. I couldn't understand most of what he said.

What bothers me the most, more than all these misunderstandings, is that he refused to let me read my list of problems. Because my hypersensitivity to sound was on there, my raging, burning diarrhea was on there. The deterioration of my handwriting and my inability to count money and do basic math was on there. How I'd lost the ability to read when the letters had started to run down the page and how I still struggled to comprehend written words with the ease I'd once had was on there.

He might've gotten a clue, but he literally cut me off when I tried to read my list. The other thing that bothers me is his note that the only reason I was seeing him was for his opinion on how to get better. I was seeing him for information. I wanted to understand every little detail of how the changes to my brain had come about. Who granted him the power to decide I shouldn't have access to information?

But let's talk about the letter I finally got from him. It said the literature since the 1900s shows that people with psychogenic movement disorder/conversion disorder have unusual responses to medications. The logical, scientific thing to do would be to investigate why that pattern of responses to medication exists among that patient population. You know? Do a systematic evaluation to determine what mechanisms might underlie that pattern, rather than assuming something that can't be measured, like mental illness, is the cause.

But I was starting to figure out that most doctors don't do logic.

*

I'd asked around online to see where I should go for another opinion. Someone I knew from college steered me toward the neurology department of a different hospital. I got an appointment for February 2015, because a neuropsychiatrist had just had a cancellation.

The PMDD was gone, but I wasn't quite happy because I was struggling with all the new problems with my brain. My body had pretty well healed from my hysterectomy, but I still had the speech, mouth movement, and cognitive challenges. They'd improved a little in the weeks following the Depo-Medrol injection but still caused major problems in my daily life.

And I had panic—terrible, terrible panic. Horror-show panic. Hide-in-the-closet panic. I was taking a benzo that Dr. Iyilik had prescribed for the anxiety, Imodium for my incessant diarrhea, prazosin for my nightmares, and an estrogen patch for hormone replacement. I only took the benzo every few days though because it made me feel sad.

I gripped the folder that held my paperwork, which included a medication list, a timeline of the onset of my symptoms, and a complete list of all of the psych drugs I'd ever taken. They also documented recent changes, like the strange sounds I now heard. Near the end of 2014, I'd begun to hear banging and other noises that seemed almost supernatural.

Of course, I'd included my concerns about my slurred and stammering speech and my abnormal mouth and movements, which seemed to be the only things neurologists wanted to acknowledge.

"Hi, I'm Dr. Anjān," the resident introduced himself. He was a clean-cut looking man with hair and skin a shade or two darker than mine. He glanced over the paperwork I offered. "I'm going to go give this to Dr. Jape for review. He'll look at it while I start your evaluation. Then he'll join us later."

When Anjān returned, he sat down and spoke. "Tell me about when you started to be depressed."

"Um, around when I was eight I think. I know I first tried to kill myself when I was eight."

"Why did you do that?"

"I was always getting beat up at school, and nobody at home cared about me."

"How was school for you academically? How far did you go?"

"I h-h-have a bachelor's degree."

The effort it was taking to understand him and respond was wearing me down.

"Did you do any drugs?"

"I tried d-d-drugs, but I didn't really like them."

"What drug was your favorite?"

"Um, I don't know. I d-did, uh, uh, acid a couple of times, so I g-g-guess I liked it." I was trying hard to give the right answers. His question told me I was supposed to have had a favorite drug. I hadn't. I'd always hated the way drugs made me feel.

"I'm sure you smoked pot, right?" He gave a little smile that made me feel dirty.

I hadn't tried pot until college. Some of my mother's boyfriends had been potheads. I'd tried to avoid any of the activities those devil men had participated in. But I knew that was the wrong answer. Anjān made it sound like everyone was supposed to have smoked pot. I didn't want to give the wrong answer to a psychiatrist. He could lock me up for the wrong answer.

"Um, I m-may have tried it, but I didn't like it," I replied after turning the question and how I should answer it over in my mind.

Anjān moved on. "You didn't pursue any education beyond a bachelor's degree?"

"Huh? Um, well I wanted to. But, um—after I got my degree, I applied to law school and g-g-got accepted. But I couldn't afford to g-go. So, I didn't go." I spoke the scripted line I'd spoken so many times before to the people who'd asked why I'd stopped at a bachelor's degree.

Anjān seemed satisfied. I thought from his suppressed smirk, slight nod, and lowered brow that he might have detected some artifice. But he was happy all the same. Of course he was happy. It was exactly as he'd expected. He'd identified my answer as an excuse and was delighted by his insight. I could imagine him considering the options. *Typical underachiever? Afraid of success. Self-sabotaging? A liar? Someone who'd had such a childhood could never amount to much. She probably never even got into law school. Yeah, that's it. She's making the whole thing up.*

His head was bobbing vigorously now. He closed his folder and stood up to go get Dr. Jape.

Another white-coated man entered the room. His broad, pale face was tinged with pink. My attention was drawn to his tie, which was illustrated with book covers. They were embellished with titles from the Bible. *Revelation* boomed the text on the spine of the largest one.

Dr. Jape asked a few more questions.

"So, you had PMDD?" he asked without requesting a definition of the acronym.

"Yes, I did until m-my hysterectomy last D-December."

"And you had ECT, but it didn't help your mood because the PMDD was hormonal?"

"Yes, exactly!"

"What problems do you think you're having now?"

"I'm having s-s-serious problems with my memory. I get really confused, especially at night. I get lost. I hardly ever drive anymore or even walk without my husband, b-because I can't f-figure out where I am half the t-time. I just can't think cl-clearly anymore. I can't do basic math, which is ridi-di-di-culous and embarrassing."

"Are you paying attention?" he asked.

*Are you serious?* I wanted to blurt. I tamped down the outburst and nodded. Then I took a breath and waited for the words to form. "Yes, I'm p-paying attention."

"What kind of car did you drive to get here? What highway did you take to get to this city?"

I wanted to explain that those weren't the types of things I had trouble remembering, but I couldn't find the words. I answered his questions correctly.

"You're seeing a gastrointestinal specialist. Were you sick as a child?" He was nodding.

"Huh? Um, well, I heard some s-s-stories from my mom that I had some kinda immune deficiency as uh, uh, a baby, but I don't know the details. My mother's really dr-dr-dramatic and she's also a l-l-liar, so I'm not sure if that's t-true." I reached into the vague memories of conversations with my mother. Her truths were as vivid as her lies, and both were spouted with equal frequency and conviction.

"Do you *remember* being sick as a young child?" Dr. Jape asked.

"Well, not really. Just some stomachaches. I faked being sick some to stay home from school, because I was always getting bullied." I didn't want to admit that I'd shit my pants until I was eleven years old.

His nods were brisk, and his eyes were narrowed.

"How's your depression now?"

"It's gone. It's been gone since the hysterectomy."

"How about your anxiety?"

"It's terrible! Unbearable, really. That's what's killing me," I blurted.

He asked me to do a series of exercises, many of the same ones Dr. Wise and Dr. Crow had asked me to do: Walk down the hall and back. Touch my finger to my nose. I kept getting confused by his instructions, but I followed them as best I could.

"This is a functional neurological disorder. It's like a malfunctioning of the software in your brain. It's caused by stress," he went on, saying some things I couldn't follow. He wrote down the address of a website for me to check out, Neurosymptoms.org. His voice was calm.

"How confident are you in this diagnosis?" piped Andrew.

"Well, like any diagnosis, it's not 100 percent. But with FND, the diagnostic error rate is less than with other neurological disorders," he said. "A leading FND researcher estimates the misdiagnosis rate at around just 5 percent."

"The good news is, I think if you get your anxiety under control, this will all go away," Dr. Jape continued. "I recommend you take Zoloft. That will make your anxiety improve, and everything else will improve along with it."

Andrew drove us home. I felt good. Dr. Jape had answered all our questions, and he'd explained things really well. He'd definitely been a better communicator than Dr. Crow, and he'd spent more time with us than Dr. Wise. But a bit of doubt persisted. *What happened to me didn't seem psychogenic, because my meditation practice didn't touch it, but maybe it somehow was.*

I was scared to take Zoloft, because the last time I'd taken it, the movement and speech problems had gotten worse, but I thought I'd give it one more shot. I was at the point with my brain problems that I'd once been at with the PMDD. I was willing to do anything to get my functioning back.

On the drive home, I pulled up Neurosymptoms.org on my phone and read about functional neurological disorder. I paused when I realized FND was an umbrella term for over thirty symptoms, and I only had a few of them. I had fatigue, sleep problems, memory and concentration challenges, word-finding difficulties, GI problems, and slurred speech.

I didn't have seizures or blackouts. And I hadn't had much pain since I'd gotten off the Lupron. I hadn't had bladder problems since the Depo-Medrol reaction, and while it often felt like there was a lot of pressure in my head, it didn't seem to be the same thing as a headache. I'd never had tremors.

What I read made me skeptical of Dr. Jape's diagnosis, but I pushed the skepticism to the back of my mind. I wanted to hold on to the most remote shred of hope that the Zoloft could help me heal.

Andrew pulled into the driveway, and my eyes were drawn to a scene transpiring at the house behind ours. An ambulance and fire engine were parked in the street, and EMTs were running in and out of the home. I tossed and turned for hours before falling asleep around midnight. I slept until four twenty-one a.m., when this happened:

*2/12/15*

*Sitting in office with door locked at 4:21am. Phone near my lap. Worst nightmare of my life ever, ever, ever. I dreamed I tried to wake up Andrew because he made a sound like he was choking. Instead of rolling over or something, he reached up and choked me. I tried to get away, running, getting choked. The dream would end and then start over and over again. One time, he woke up and I knew he was going to choke me so I ran outside, trying to scream for help but I couldn't make any sounds. Trying to get to a neighbor. Knowing I wasn't going* to make it. *The dream kept repeating. I got into a neighbor's house and was trying to hide, and he was trying to beat down the door. That woke me up. I'm in the office now. It was so horrifyingly real I'm scared beyond explanation. I wish I could talk to someone. When I am most scared, I talk to him but I'm scared of him. I am so scared that on some level this is real. Things in the world have been strange. Left the most encouraging doctor appointment but everything seems like a strange and scary sign. Phone died for first time ever in the car on the way back from Missouri and refused hard reboot. Sakari [husky] tried to sleep right beside me in bed. She never does that. I feel absolutely horrified and fucking crazy right now. I'm fucking scared to death. He has never touched me in a mean way, but I am so scared and this is so real that maybe he could snap and become as crazy as me and try to kill me. I have no idea how to get through this. I think his alarm is set for 5:00, it's 4:27. I hope he wakes up at 5 and is normal. I'm scared to go back to sleep. But I'm exhausted. Is this a sleep deprivation nightmare? I took 2 mg prazosin. But I couldn't sleep. Then the emergency crews came to the house behind us. Bad pre-sleep influence? Even with all the panic I have had since my surgery, this is the very worst thing to happen ever. I'm so scared, and it seemed so real I am almost dialing 911. But he is in bed asleep. And I feel uninjured. It must have been a dream. This room is locked. It would take him a long time to find the right key. I'm still scared to go to sleep. I can't go to sleep. I must sit here until he wakes up and I confirm he is normal, himself, harmless.*

 *5:40, still awake. His alarm just went off. He did not get up.*
 *5:50 2<sup>nd</sup> alarm.*

 I'd typed those words on that terrifying morning. At around six a.m., Andrew came looking for me. He knocked on the office door. After some discussion through the door, I let him in. When he opened the door, I realized the scene had been a dream. I'd had vivid dreams for years, but I usually recognized when I was dreaming. Sometimes, I could even force myself to wake up or take control of the dream. This time had been different. I'd been completely unable to distinguish the dream from reality long after I'd awoken.

Andrew drove me to my appointment with Grace that afternoon. I handed her the sheet I'd typed about the hallucination.

"Don't you see that's you!" she exclaimed. "That's not Andrew in your dream! That's you. You're afraid of yourself."

"I was thinking it might have been because she stopped taking her Ativan," Andrew said. "She didn't know you can't cold turkey quit a benzodiazepine, you have to taper off. She'd been taking it every day for a couple of weeks this time, and then she'd quit because it was making her feel sad."

"Well, maybe," Grace conceded. "But I still think dreams have meaning. And I think she was the attacker in the dream, not you."

I knew she was wrong, but I couldn't form speech that day to correct her.

"Before you went to see this new neurologist, you said your anxiety was out of control. Why won't you take your meds?" Grace asked.

"I. Hate. B-b-benzos," I tried.

"But you're sick! You have to take your meds! You have a brain illness. You have to take your meds!" she insisted.

I sat back, closed my eyes, and shook my head.

"How'd the appointment go?" Grace transitioned.

"Good," Andrew answered. "We got good news from the doctor. He thinks she has something called functional neurological disorder, and that if her anxiety gets controlled by Zoloft, all of her other symptoms will go away."

I nodded. Letters, like glowing Scrabble tiles, danced in my head.

"That's great!" Grace cheered. "How was the drive?"

"The roads were clear. We had lots of great conversation. On the way home, she told me all about Malcolm X and the different black advocacy movements of the 1960s," Andrew said.

"Malcolm X?" Grace repeated with a small chuckle.

"Yes, seriously," Andrew said. He'd heard the laugh in her voice too and didn't understand why Malcolm X was a humorous topic.

"Well, okay," said Grace. She turned to me. "Why can't you talk? You got good news! Why can't you talk?"

I shook my head. I didn't know why. My ears hurt. My brain hurt. I was exhausted.

"You got good news!" she insisted. "Talk! I don't understand why you can't talk when you got good news! Come on, talk!"

The sounds from the bathroom adjacent to Grace's office stormed through my brain. *Flush, clang, bang, slam!* I opened my mouth to try to explain but could only conjure breath.

"You got good news. Talk!" she urged again.

I began to cry. I wanted to talk. I wanted to think. But I couldn't do either.

"Okay," she said. "Well, go home, take your meds, and get some sleep. Maybe then you'll be able to talk."

***

**Grace laughing about Malcolm X. Did that offend you?**

Offend? No. It just revealed more about her. It sealed a pattern. On any of the rare occasions I'd tried to talk to her about how race affected me, like how some people treated me badly because I'm black or brown or mixed or whatever, she'd just look at me and say, "Isn't everyone mixed?" Then she'd give me that therapist stare while I sat there thinking, *You are truly clueless, aren't you?*

You know what I mean? There's white people, mostly older ones, who think that race is a social construct. Well, yeah it is. Of course it is. But then they make this mental leap that social construct somehow magically translates to *we should all just realize we're the same and lean in for a big 'ol homogenous hug,* like acknowledging that race is a social construct is gonna wipe out hundreds of years of racial bias and discrimination in the United States. Like I can say, "Oh, everybody's mixed," and that'll keep the Klan types from treating me like a piece of shit.

I'd been down that road before, and it always turned out the same way. People start talking over me. I get overwhelmed and become silent. Then whomever I'm arguing with walks away thinking they've won, or convinced me that I'm wrong, or that I don't have a defense or whatever—just because I've never been able to hold my own in a spoken argument.

# CHAPTER TWENTY-THREE

LET ME CATCH you up on how the whole GI thing was going. Soa was a physician assistant, remember? Well, her supervising doctor had done a colonoscopy back in October of '14 and had told me everything looked fine. I'd looked at the pictures, and my colon had looked all yellow and inflamed, but what did I know?

I'd switched to another doctor, Dr. Moon. He'd done another colonoscopy a few weeks after my first one, and he'd removed two polyps that Soa's buddy had missed. Moon also did an endoscopy. He'd told me that both had showed inflammation.

I went back to Dr. Moon because I was having excruciating abdominal pain and watery diarrhea all day long. I couldn't leave the house because it was so bad.

I walked to the check-in counter, which was divided into two sections. The right side housed a receptionist for gastroenterology patients, and the left side housed a receptionist for neurosurgery. As I was waiting for the receptionist to scan my driver's license and insurance card, a tall, round man stepped up to the neurosurgery counter.

"What's your name, sir?" asked the receptionist.

"Frank McGillicuddy!" the man boomed.

The receptionist paused. "Could you spell that, please?"

"Bwaaaaa! It's a joke! Ha-ha-ha-ha! I'm Steve Jones! I'm more Archie Bunker than Frank McGillicuddy," he said as he shot a cold look in my direction.

I ran from the counter to escape the man's voice. But the opposite side of the room had a squawking television on the wall. I reached in my purse for earbuds. I touched an icon to drown out the sounds with my white noise app, but I couldn't get a signal.

I darted away from the TV. The shouting man had finally stepped away from the desk. I saw five empty chairs against a wall of windows. I plopped down on the last chair in the row. I hoped that the other chairs stayed empty. But as soon as I thought this, a woman with bleached-blond hair and black roots and two shrieking, barefoot kids plopped into the chairs. Trailing behind her was a sleeveless man with a shaved head. He carried a screaming infant. The children's wails, and the smells of sweat, hamburger grease, and nicotine raced into my ears and up my nostrils. My stomach churned.

I rose to my feet and ran. "I n-n-need my driver's license! I have to g-g-go," I stuttered as I shoved the clipboard with the partially completed paperwork at the receptionist.

"What?" The young man gazed at me.

"Give me my shit! I have t-to leave!" I cried.

I turned to run the second the cards were in my hands. I found my car and shifted into reverse. I pulled out of my space and began to look for the exit. Around and around I drove, but I couldn't find the tollbooth.

I pulled into a parking spot and turned off the engine. I tried to text Andrew, but I still couldn't get a signal. I headed back into the building, hoping I'd get service once I left the garage.

I texted: *It's loud. I'm confused. Can't think. Help please.*

*I'm at work. What do you want me to do?* I read the words and began to cough. The coughing turned to sobs that stuck in my throat.

I wandered the corridors in search of quiet. The beige hallways all looked the same. Tears streamed as I stumbled forward. I passed dozens of people in scrubs and white coats, but no one seemed to see me.

Andrew's texts rolled in. *Where are you?* I typed back, *In the building.* I tried to focus on my breath and reach for clarity, but all I heard was noise—voices, footfalls, equipment beeps, elevator chimes, clanging carts. I did my best to avert my eyes from motion, because the spinning wheels of the carts and the flashes of light would suck me in, paralyzing my attention and immobilizing my body.

*Ask someone for directions*, the text said.

Figures zipped past me. Fear coursed through me at the thought of speaking to any of them. I backed into a corner and slid down the wall. I buried my face in my hands and began to wail. My ears were on fire. My head was going to explode.

"Err ooh Tie lah?"

The voice repeated, "Are you Twilah?"

I looked up. A man in a blue uniform loomed before me. *Oh shit. I'm going to get shot now. This is where it ends.*

I saw Gautama, the Buddha. I thought about the bardo, the in-between state where the consciousness goes after death. I had to be ready.

"Your husband sent me to find you," the uniform said. I could barely understand his words.

Husband? I stood and followed the blue man. After what felt like hours winding through the labyrinthine corridors of the hospital, I saw Andrew. I fell into his arms and closed my eyes.

❧

**Did you ever reschedule with Dr. Moon?**

Nope. Wasn't worth it. I was having accidents at that point, but I just decided to live with the poop and the pain.

# CHAPTER TWENTY-FOUR

I'D APPLIED FOR Social Security Disability benefits in July 2013, way before I'd known I could get a hysterectomy that would cure the PMDD. By July, I'd realized there was no way the PMDD would allow me to work.

The first Social Security Disability Insurance (SSDI) denial had been in December 2013. After the letter had come, I'd looked into hiring an attorney. I'm not a big fan of legal representation for things like that, because in insurance it's well known that most attorneys don't do anything other than take a huge percentage of the same settlement the claimant would've been offered anyway. But I knew my brain was too messed up for me to be able to represent myself.

In 2014, I'd filled out contact forms with a couple of firms, and within hours, Dick Grede with Grede and Associates had called me. He'd assured me he'd fight for my case. "Okay." I'd assented to the words I could barely understand.

A few days later, Andrew and I met with one of Grede's associates in the Kansas City office. I don't remember the meeting with the attorney, Cindy Clutchfield, at all. Andrew tells me she was cold and short with us.

I did everything the law firm asked me to do. I kept logs of my doctor and therapy appointments, and I sent the logs in every three weeks. Except once.

It was in June 2014. You know, when I was still getting ECT. The firm had sent me a packet to fill out, and I'd put it in a drawer and forgotten about it. I vaguely remembered a woman from Grede calling me and asking me about the packet. When she'd called, she'd woken me up, and I'd been really disoriented.

She'd spent less than five minutes asking me questions. And later, I don't know, maybe a few weeks later, I'd gotten another denial letter from Social Security. I hadn't realized the lady from Grede had been calling for information on which they were going to base my appeal.

In August 2014, I called Grede to explain my new neurological problems. My assigned paralegal, a woman named Ohdyiss, took my call.

"Um, hi, um. My name's Twilah Hiari, and I, um, am calling because I have a n-n-ew diagnosis."

"You don't need to call us with this. Everything'll be in your file. Your attorney will know everything when it's time for your hearing," she snapped. After asking for repetition, I finally understood her.

In January 2015, I'd received a packet of paperwork from Social Security. But I couldn't make sense of the documents.

"Grede Law Firm," a woman answered.

"Yes, I have a c-c-case pending, and I need h-h-elp completing some pap-er-erwork I just got from Social Security."

The receptionist took my information and transferred me to a paralegal. I stammered out a short voicemail message.

Two days later, my phone rang. "This is Ohdyiss with Grede Law returning your call. How can I help you?" asked the woman.

"I got th-this packet from Social Security, and I'm n-n-ot sure how they want it f-f-filled out. I was hoping you'd h-h-help me."

"Just follow the directions," she snapped.

"Huh?" Silence hung between us until I'd reviewed her words and understood them. "I, I, I'm trying. I sent you all this stuff already. Can't you just send your copies to Social S-S-Security for me? Or can I just p-print the doctor stuff off m-my in-insurance company's website and send it in? I can't understand t-th-these forms. Ima, Ima, Ima having tr-trouble writing."

"It's not that hard. Just fill it out and send it back. Are you still at your same address?" she interrupted and said my current address.

"Yes," I responded after a long pause I needed to understand her.

"Well, I have to ask. Our clients never stay put, they're all over the place, and we can't get in touch with them half the time—blah-blah-blah," she complained. "Just fill out the paperwork, and call us when you have a hearing date."

*Well, when you have no income to pay your rent or mortgage, that might put you in a position where you have to move a lot, you stupid bitch.* My throat was jammed with a thick black clot of rage. I swallowed it and spoke.

"Also, I no longer have PMDD, which is the o-o-or-r-r-iginal reason I applied for disability. I'm having n-n-neurological problems now—so should I get another medical s-s-source statement since I have a different disability th-than I had b-b-before?"

"No! More is not better. Don't think more is better, blah-blah-blah," she said. "Just fill out the forms and send them back."

"Y-y-you know, if I could fill out these f-f-forms, I could pr-probably work. But I c-c-can't. I need your help."

"Just do your best."

In April 2015, I learned that a hearing had been scheduled with an administrative law judge. I called Grede Law and asked for Ohdyiss. The person who answered told me she was no longer with the firm. I was transferred to voicemail. Two days later, I was still waiting for my call to be returned. I called again and was transferred to a different paralegal after I demanded to speak to a supervisor.

"This is Termagant," a woman answered.

"Uh, hi, Tur—what's your name?" I said.

"This is TERM-A-GANT," she repeated loudly.

"Hi, um, I have a hearing coming up, and I want to make s-s-sure everything's ready."

The sigh in my ear was painful. "I'll call you for a phone conference when it gets closer to your hearing date. You don't need to call us!"

"Um, is there any way I can m-m-meet with someone instead of having a ph-ph-phone conference? Phone c-c-calls are really, really hard f-f-for me."

"Well, I'm two hundred miles away in Rolla, Missouri. What do you expect me to do?" she countered.

"Can I meet with s-s-somebody in Kansas City?"

"That's not the way we do it. But if you're that special, maybe I can get you an appointment down there."

"T-t-that would be good. Do y-y-you have an evening appointment? I get confused and lost, s-s-so I try not to drive anymore," I said. Andrew had exhausted his time off and was at risk of being fired for unplanned absences. "I n-n-need my husband to t-t-take me when he gets off work."

"No. We're open from eight to five. I don't know what to tell you," she said with another sigh.

"You f-f-fucking know what? For a firm that stands to earn $6,000 from my m-m-medical misfortune, you really can't tell me shit," I said. "Can I t-t-talk to my attorney?"

"Sure, I'll have her call you." Termagant hung up.

Twenty minutes later, my phone rang.

"Hello, this is your attorney, Cindy Clutchfield. You wanted to speak to me?"

I pulled the microphone of my earbuds closer to my mouth. "Y-y-yes. Given the course of interactions with your firm over the past year, I have z-z-zero confidence in your ability to represent me. I would like s-s-some degree of assurance that my counsel is remotely within the realm of c-c-competence," I raged.

"Ooh, that sounded good. Did you read that off of a script?" she shot back.

I took a breath and unclenched my teeth. Cindy had graduated from a fourth-tier law school. I'm sure she knew a lot about reading off of scripts.

"D-d-id I read that off a script? Are you fucking s-s-serious right now?"

"Your speech is slurred; did you take your meds?"

"My sp-sp-speech is fucked up because I have a neurological disorder that I told your firm about f-f-fucking months ago. I n-n-no longer want to be represented by you. Send me t-t-termination papers, and s-s-send me my file."

"Let me get you back to Termagant to discuss your prehearing paperwork packet." She dropped me back into the phone queue.

"It might take a few weeks to get you a CD of your file," said Termagant when she picked up.

"That's n-n-not acceptable. I want it n-n-next week so I can get new representation," I seethed.

"Well, that's not in my control."

I collapsed on the futon in my office and held Sakari, wiping my tears onto the husky's fur. Then I typed out a letter to Dick Grede. I delineated my experience with Clutchfield and the paralegals at his firm. I asked that I not be billed for any services. I never received a response to my letter.

---

**You'd gotten caught up in a cycle of exploitation?**

It felt like I was caught in a Kafka novel. Mill after mill. The medical mill chewed me up and spit me out. The disability law mill did the same. I'll mention though, while we're on the subject of lawyers, that Andrew had contacted a few of them to talk about malpractice after Dr. Wise had given me the tardive dyskinesia diagnosis. And none of them were remotely interested in taking my case. They didn't come out and say it, but I think it might be because I'd make a bad witness. You know? Because I'd been a long-term psych patient. I mean, that's fine now, because TD wasn't truly what I'd had. I would've lost the case, because I didn't have TD. But the clock was ticking on a malpractice or product liability suit.

***It's almost like every professional had turned against you at that point.***

Huh? Yeah, it seemed that way. That's the power of diagnostic overshadowing. Once you're perceived as mentally ill, all bets are off. I'm not gonna lie. This was the worst time in my entire life—worse than the abuse when I was a kid, worse than the PMDD.

I mean, I knew something had messed up my brain. I couldn't speak right or speak at all half the time, and I kept getting told that it was all in my head, that it was somehow within my control. Ha-ha, like my brain's not in my head.

It was like all the rest of the lies I'd been told. These professionals were trying to tell me that up was down, that reality was something other than what it was. It was like something out of science fiction. But you know, nothing lasts forever. Nothing. Except for misdiagnoses, I guess.

"My God, honey. I could just fall down and sleep on the sidewalk," I said. "That's not hyperbole. I can't make my body move anymore."

"We're only a mile from home. You can make it," Andrew encouraged.

"I, I, I dunno." Every cell in my body felt like it was grinding to a halt.

Andrew stopped and looked at me. "Oh. You don't look so good. At all. You're pale. Stay here, and I'll go home and get the car."

"Oka-a-a-y." Minutes later, I was asleep on the park bench.

It was June 2015. I'd been taking Zoloft for almost five months, and my anxiety was worse than it had been when Dr. Jape had recommended the drug. My speech was still messed up. My mouth and jaw were moving around all crazy again. I was in a constant state of confusion. My short-term memory was a little better, but not close to what it had once been.

In the months since I'd seen Dr. Jape, I'd done a lot of reading on functional neurological disorder. And I was becoming more and more convinced that it didn't apply to me. I could go for a full-day retreat at the Buddhist temple across the street from a fire station and be in blissful meditation right up to the moment a fire truck turned on its siren—then I'd become anxious and confused. Before 2014, I hadn't liked the sirens from the station, but I could quickly resume my focus after the disruption. Now, almost all sound resulted in complete mental disintegration.

Beyond realizing that a functional or psychogenic hypothesis was wrong for me, I'd realized it was a bullshit diagnosis for anyone. It was a handy little blame-the-victim bucket.

It works like this: A neurologist does the usual brief office exam, maybe even orders a brain MRI. Neither the exam nor the MRI show any abnormalities that correspond to a diagnosis in the canon of known neurological disorders. So, the neurologist throws up his hands and says, "I don't see anything, so it must be psychological." Mind you, he doesn't have any affirmative evidence that it's psychological, but he has the power to make the diagnosis anyway. He sends the patient to a shrink, and the shrink gives the patient psych drugs. The drugs don't do shit to help the situation and sometimes make the symptoms worse.

And if FND is psychogenic or due to trauma, why wasn't it more prevalent in survivors of major conflicts? Why weren't its symptoms ever mentioned in slave narratives, historical war memoirs, or incarceration memoirs? There had to be other variables at work.

I'll tell you something else about the FND diagnosis that was a big red flag: The misdiagnosis rate is allegedly 5 percent, like Dr. Jape had said. But it isn't clear whether that 5 percent only includes people who were later found to have different *neurological* diagnoses. You see what I mean? Does it include people who have illnesses that are later found to originate in other body systems but present neurologically?

I chatted with lots of people in FND forums. And there were *lots* of people who had been misdiagnosed. Some people turned out to have diseases I'd never heard of—rare neurological, endocrine, or autoimmune diseases, sometimes even cardiac disorders. How well do you think neurologists, especially older neurologists, are trained to recognize these diseases? And shrinks too? I mean, how many immune, autoimmune, or endocrine disorders with psychiatric manifestations can you name? Do you see how there's a serious issue with how Western medicine is so siloed, so hyperspecialized?

And I wondered how many people were misdiagnosed but had given up—the ones who had completely disengaged after one too many episodes of abuse from the medical profession. The ones who were like, "Well, it's FND, and there's no help. It's all in my head, and I'm screwed." I chatted with people who said they'd rather sit at home in excruciating pain than get treated like a drug seeker by nurses and physicians. And where are misdiagnosed people supposed to report their misdiagnoses? How do you even get included in the 5 percent figure?

I decided to try to visit one more neurologist. Guess I'm a fucking optimist.

In the lobby of Bourgie Neurology, signs posted on the walls and doors said *Audio and Video Recording Prohibited.*

Exhaustion overtook me, and I dozed off to the sound of white noise piping through my earbuds. Over an hour after my scheduled appointment time, I woke up to the sound of a woman yelling a mispronounced version of my name. I followed her to an exam room where she explained the facility's billing policy. Before they'd perform any tests, they wanted a thousand dollars up front.

"B-but you verified my insurance and that I have $1,300 in my health reimbursement account," I said.

"Doesn't matter. We need $1,000 before running any tests," she repeated.

Two hours after my scheduled appointment time, a man entered the room. "I'm Dr. Bamstick!" His chest expanded as he roared his name. "This is my nurse, Bob!"

Bamstick continued, booming, "I looked at your records. You had this menstrual depression disorder!"

"It's called p-premenstrual dysphoric d-disorder. PMDD," I corrected him.

"Yeah. So, you had this menstrual depression disorder and you have PTSD too?" he continued.

"I had PTSD, yes, though it's mostly r-r-resolved. I still have a few triggers, but it's way better than it used to be. I have anxiety, but I don't think it's from the PTSD. The PMDD is gone. It was c-c-cured by a hysterectomy last December."

"Why do you have PTSD? Were you in the service?" He gave me a skeptical look.

"Um, no. It's from childhood trauma."

"Oh. What did your parents do? Punch you and kick you?" he blurted. "Huh? Did they? Punch you and kick you?"

My silence in that moment had nothing to do with my speech or auditory issues. I was frozen in a netherworld between fight and flight.

"Huh? What was it? Punching you and kicking you? Did they throw you up against walls?"

I shook my head slowly. My eyes were wide.

"Did they? Huh? Throw you against walls? What did they do to you?" he shouted.

I sat silent. Frozen. Terrified.

"Whatever then," he declared once he'd realized I wasn't going to answer. "Take off your shoes."

"Um, my husband usually c-comes to my appointments with me. He couldn't come today because he didn't have any time off left. Can I c-call him and put him on sp-speakerphone?"

"No!" Nurse Bob and Dr. Bamstick shouted in unison.

My tears flowed. My shoes dropped to the floor with small thuds. Bamstick took an instrument and stroked it over the sole of my right foot.

"Clowem us! Mild!" he barked at the nurse, who was typing on a laptop. "Hypurr Eflexia! Blah-blah-blah . . ."

I don't remember much about the rest of the appointment. A woman came in and gave me a short test called the Montreal Cognitive Assessment.

"You seriously don't remember?" she'd spat the words at me with a roll of her eyes when I'd been unable to repeat any of the words she'd told me to memorize.

Dr. Bamstick ordered a sleep study, a cervical MRI, and an EEG.

"My sister-in-law is a sleep tech, and I want her to d-do the study," I told the scheduler.

"No," she said. "We need everything done in-house. We need to know that the person reading the study knows what they're doing. If you make that payment of a thousand dollars, I'll schedule you right now."

"Um, let me talk to m-my husband, and we'll c-call back," I murmured.

Dr. Bamstick and Associates had made Dr. Crow seem like the king of affability. There were clearly no behaviorally based interviews for neurology hires. I tried to think of other professions where these types of interactions might be acceptable. *Interrogator at Guantanamo? Supermax prison guard? Drill sergeant for ISIS recruits?*

My health was in these people's hands. My tears had been dried by the rising heat of rage.

*What had Bamstick said about my feet?* I asked myself. With help from Dr. Google, I determined the words had been *clonus* and *hyperreflexia. What caused those things?*

Octopus poisoning and kuru, a prion disease caused by cannibalism, were among the causes Dr. Google reported. Those didn't fit my diet, I realized with a small laugh. *Thanks again, Dr. Google. You helped me rule out a couple of more problems, and you didn't make me cry.* I was becoming enlightened to the madness of medicine. I knew I needed to distance myself from it to maintain the sanity doctors didn't believe I had.

One of the farmers I worked for at the market each summer invited me to lunch.

"Hi!" Tracy said as she took her place at the table across from me. "How have you been?"

"I, I, I've b-b-been g-g-good," I lied. I felt the left side of my lower lip pulling down.

"Let's ask for a table outside—where it's quieter," she suggested.

On the patio, a big umbrella shielded us from the glare of the sun. The unseasonably cool air had deterred other diners from requesting seating in the area.

"Is this better?" Tracy asked me once we were settled.

"Wow, yes!" My speech had instantly become clearer. The odd lip movement had become less pronounced.

Tracy smiled. "My grandson's like that. You know—Robert? The one with autism? He can't think when it's noisy. We went to McDonald's the other day after his therapy appointment. There was a sports team in there having lunch. Robert walked in, turned around, and walked right back out. I asked him why he'd left. He said it had been too loud. This is great anyway. I love the fresh air."

We talked about quilting over plates of crepes and fruit. Later, I considered how my brain had responded to the quiet. I also thought about how when I'd met Robert at the farmers market, I'd been struck by how my behavior as a child had looked a lot like his.

---

**When you realized that your behavior as a young person looked like Robert's, did you wonder if you might be autistic?**

Well, yeah, for like a minute, then I rejected the idea. I second-guessed myself because my thought process was, *Well, I acted like that at his age, but over time I'd stopped engaging in some of those behaviors, even if some of those behaviors have come back.* I thought that autism is a lifelong, completely unchangeable condition. Therefore, I concluded, what I was experiencing couldn't be autism.

Which is ridiculous—I mean, when I started to read about autism, like really dig in to the literature, I didn't find a single study that had lasted for more than twenty years! The majority of autistic people my age and older are of the Asperger's variety, and didn't get diagnosed until adulthood. Or they're still undiagnosed.

And you know, for some people that's fine. It might not add any value to their lives. But think of the people in psych wards and mental health offices who are getting called bipolar or borderline, people who are getting called persistent failures by therapists because they can't conform to neurotypical behaviors. People who've been missing that mark—that therapist-created goal—for twenty or thirty years now. For those people, it's a big goddamned problem!

Can I have a tissue please? I get really upset over this. It's personal. It really touches me. Let me take a breath here. But think about what I said. A physicist can give you a good description of what something will look like in the future based on formulas and calculations. A psychologist or therapist, not so much. Humans don't work like that.

# CHAPTER TWENTY-FIVE

GRACE, DR. IYILIK, and I had all reached out to Dr. Jape to try to get the records from my visit, but Dr. Jape hadn't responded to any of us. Finally, after I fired Grede Law, my new attorney sent Dr. Jape a letter requesting the record. The attorney's letter had prompted Dr. Jape to complete his report in July 2015, five months after he saw me. And what a diagnosis it was!

> Somatization disorder: Her history is very suggestive of Briquet's syndrome, but available history does not confirm it.
> Atypical dystonia: The mouth and speech problems are most consistent with a functional neurological problem. The timing essentially rules out tardive dystonia, and the phenomenology is atypical anyway. Amitriptyline does not cause TD (although like any anticholinergic, it can worsen pre-existing TD).
> Depression: recurrent major depression: 296.35 The PT

feels her depression is gone, but she barely misses criteria for a current episode.
Anxiety disorder NOS: Mixed anxiety disorder with panic, agoraphobia and PTSD features. [A/P late entry 08 July 2015 from notes 2/11/2015]

Briquet's syndrome, according to a page from Brown University, is described as a condition where "patients feel that they have been sickly most of their lives and complain of a multitude of symptoms referable to numerous different organ systems. This conviction of illness persists despite repeatedly negative and unrevealing consultations, hospitalizations, and diagnostic procedures, and patients continue to seek medical care, to take prescription medications, and to submit to needless diagnostic procedures."

The DSM IV criteria for Somatization disorder are:

> A history of somatic complaints over several years, starting prior to age of thirty.
> Such symptoms cannot be fully explained by a general medical condition or substance use OR, when there is an associated medical condition, the impairments due to the somatic symptoms are more severe than generally expected. Complaints are not feigned as in malingering or factitious disorder.

*❧*

***Dr. Jape thought it was all in your head and always had been?***
Yeah. And psychiatry had invented a diagnosis to blame the patient for the diagnostic shortcomings of modern medicine: Somatization. Jesus Christ!

I mean because all those positive C. diff lab results were fabrications of my sick mind. And the bronchitis and abscess that led to the antibiotics that made me susceptible to the C. diff—those were make believe too. And the known side effect of arthralgia with the Lupron was due to my lunacy. And the PMDD was a figment of my fucking demented imagination. It just happened to be magically cured by a hysterectomy. And the pathology report after my hysterectomy that showed endometriosis and fibroids in my uterus and cysts on my right ovary? I snuck into the pathology lab and made that shit up, right? Because I'm that goddamned nuts.

But that isn't even the worst part. I mean, the worst part, in my opinion, is how he put this Briquet's in my records with this caveat "available history does not confirm it." If it's not confirmed, then why's it in my medical record? And barely misses the criteria for depression? And most people a few months out from a brain injury are fucking happy?

The injury had altered my memory, my concentration, my hearing, and my speech. It'd made me bang my head against the wall like I was three years old again; like there shouldn't be a little bit of grieving when something like that happens. Imagine having all that happen, having all those losses, and then having a bunch of fucking doctors tell you that not only did it happen because you're nuts, but that you shouldn't be grieving your losses. Take a second to imagine how that felt.

---

I'd gone online and learned that the judge presiding over my hearing approved fewer SSDI cases than any other judge in the state.

I sat between Andrew and my attorney. I leaned forward in my chair and focused on the judge's lips as he spoke.

"How did the PMDD affect you before your hysterectomy?" he asked.

"Um, it made me suicidal every t-two weeks," I answered after I'd paused to process his words.

He asked several questions about the onset of my cognitive problems. Some I could answer, some I couldn't, because I was unable to remember the sequence of events. My attorney offered answers he extracted from the pile of medical records before him.

"Are there lawsuits pending against any of the physicians who treated you?" The judge's voice echoed through the courtroom.

"I'm sorry, I didn't understand. Would you repeat the question please?" My face reddened.

He repeated the question.

"No," I replied.

"What's the biggest trigger for your confusion?"

"I'm sorry, sir, would you repeat the question?"

"What is the biggest trigger for your confusion?"

"Sound."

"Sound," he repeated. "That isn't what I was expecting you to say."

A few months later, I received a letter that reported the judge's decision as fully favorable. That meant I'd be considered disabled back to the date I'd originally become disabled by the PMDD. The income from SSDI would pull our heads above water. We could pay off the new medical bills that had accrued since the bankruptcy and start to save money again.

Grede Law had had sent a bill for more than $2,000. I wrote a letter to the judge explaining my experience with Grede. The judge ordered Grede's fees to be cut in half.

*Things were looking up?*

A little, I guess. It wasn't exactly a coup to be on disability, but it was a step toward getting more financial resources so that I could figure out what the hell was going on with my brain. I hoped that if I could figure that out, I could get the hell back off of disability.

# CHAPTER TWENTY-SIX

DR. WISE'S EYES gave him an aura of quiet intelligence. He sat on his small black stool and regarded me.

"How have you been?" he asked.

I shrugged. "Pretty much the same, but more tired. I can't stay awake for more than a few hours at a time. It's irritating. I can't get anything done because I'm always exhausted or sleeping. I'll go for a walk and literally feel like I could collapse and sleep on the sidewalk. Also, I, um, had some genetic testing done, and I have this Gs152 mutation and some other mutations. I found out I'm a CYP2C19 slow metabolizer. You know? Any medication that goes through that pathway, I have a hard time breaking down."

I opened my notebook and struggled to decipher my list. "I've tried tons of drugs whose metabolism involves that pathway. Abilify, amitriptyline, Effexor, Celexa, Lexapro, Prozac, Wellbutrin, Zoloft, hell, even marijuana. I've had adverse reactions to all of them."

Dr. Wise nodded and wrote some notes in my chart. His eyes were sharp but not unkind. "Interesting. May I have a copy of these genetic results?" he asked.

"Sure, take this copy." I handed it to him.

"May I take a look at you?" he asked.

"Sure," I consented.

He performed his usual battery of exams—light in my eyes, requests to follow his instruments with my gaze. I could feel my eyes flitting about. It was hard to hold my gaze as he instructed. I thought of my meditation practice and focused on my breathing to ground my body and mind. The practice didn't stop the flitting.

"Your speech is clearer, but you still have the mouth movement," Dr. Wise stated.

"Yeah." I nodded. "I just ignore it. It's a part of me now, I guess. I saw a few other neurologists about it. They said it was psychogenic, but I don't think that's true. My mood is so much better since my hysterectomy, except for my anxiety. I don't know if it's still the PTSD or what. I mean, I don't think it's PTSD, because my nightmares and flashbacks are gone. My depression's gone too, but this anxiety is ridiculous."

"I don't think this is psychogenic," Dr. Wise said. "I can see why they went in that direction, but I don't agree that this is somatoform. I stand by my diagnosis. What else is going on?"

"I'm still really confused a lot of the time. My short-term memory is still awful, though it's a little better than it was a few months ago. At least I don't forget I put my dogs in the backyard anymore. And I don't get scared by the sound of my teapot. But I still can't do simple math at all. And I can't reason nearly as well as I used to. Reading anything of any complexity is impossible. I still get lost going to familiar places. Sometimes I go out, forget where I'm going, and end up just driving and driving. Or I end up wandering if I'm walking. I wanted to walk to the park the other day, and I ended up a couple of miles in another direction. That scared my husband real bad. I have what feels like sleep attacks. It's ridiculous really . . ." I trailed off.

"I'd like you to have a DaTScan. It will show whether the medications affected your basal ganglia, which is the center of movement. I'd also like for you to have a sleep study and neuropsychological testing to learn more about your sleep and your cognition."

"Great. I'd love to have some answers."

"You should be contacted by next week to set up those appointments. You can follow up with me after those tests are complete, in about three months. It was good seeing you again."

"Sounds good, thanks. It was good s-s-seeing you."

*Did you feel like you'd made a mistake in your assessment of Dr. Wise?*

Well, yes and no. I mean, I still thought his defense of Dr. Thueban in my records was bullshit, but I also realized it was in my best interest to move beyond that issue. Dr. Wise was the only neurologist I'd seen who was capable of rational thought and methodical inquiry. He's the only one who investigated my concerns instead of just calling me crazy.

My biggest mistake was when I'd let Soa provoke doubts in me about Dr. Wise's competence. If that hadn't happened, I would've never gone to the other neurologists who were so terrible. It turns out Dr. Wise wasn't quite right, but I don't think he was negligent either. He used all the first-line resources in his toolbox to come up with the most accurate diagnosis he could, based on the information he had at the time he saw me.

The problem is he's a neurologist, so he only had a neurology toolbox. He knew when to refer me for sleep, for neuropsych testing, and for diagnostic imaging. But he didn't know when to refer me for audiology or immunology. I don't think he knew what kind of toolbox doctors in those other specialties have—that some of them might have tools that would benefit me. But it wasn't just him; not a single other doctor thought to refer me there either.

"Hi, this is Blah from Dr. Wise's blah. I'm calling to explain blah to blah your sleep study," he said. I plugged in my earbuds and painstakingly took down the information he gave me. When I called the number he'd given me, a woman answered with what I guessed was the name of the practice. I'd noticed it was much harder to understand female voices than male voices.

"Hi, I'm calling to schedule a sleep study," I said.

"You can't just call and schedule a study. It doesn't work like that. It's not something you just walk in and do! You have to be seen by the doctor first!" she shrieked.

"I'm sorry?" I could hear anger, but there was a lag as the letters of the words she'd spoken slowly formed in my mind.

"You can't just walk in and get a study! You have to be seen first!" she raged.

"Okay," I said after taking a breath. Why was she yelling? I was just calling to schedule like I'd been told to do. "M-maybe you can explain the process to me."

"Well, you have to be seen first! Are you willing to do that?" Her voice was challenging.

"Yes! I'm willing to do whatever is protocol to have a sleep study performed. Can we start that p-process please?" I was slowly shaking my head.

Apparently, my response had finally been correct, because she managed to get me on the schedule. She was in a hurry to get off the phone now, but I stopped her. "Would you tell me the name of the doctor I'm seeing? An address would be helpful too. I was just given this number by Dr. Wise's office and told to call for a study. I don't know where I'm going or who I'm seeing."

I picked out bits and pieces of her response, "*She's the best*, and *this is her specialty*. Blah-blah-blah-blah." I still couldn't understand the doctor's name. I pressed end and typed the date into the calendar on my laptop.

At the appointment, a young blonde took my blood pressure and pulse. She was wearing a nametag, but it didn't denote her education or position.

"Why are you here today?" she asked.

"Um, I'm having problems with exhaustion and sleep attacks.

Like, I'm always tired, but sometimes I fall asleep in the middle of doing things."

"Do you have any other health issues?"

"Uh, post-infectious irritable bowel from refractory C. diff in 2014. And Dr. Wise across the way diagnosed me with tardive dyskinesia subsequent to an amitriptyline overdose," I said.

"Oh my! How did that happen?"

I gave a brief summary of how I'd been poisoned by Dr. Thueban. Her eyes grew wide. "What hospital was that at?" she asked.

"This one." I gestured with my head across the parking lot in the direction of Local Hospital.

Her brows rose. "Are you still depressed?" she asked.

"No, my depression was directly related to my hormones, and it was cured by a hysterectomy in 2014."

"What other illnesses do you have?"

"That's all."

She narrowed her eyes and looked back at her screen. "Are you sure?"

"Yes," I responded as I pressed my brows down. What an odd question.

"It says here you have post-traumatic stress disorder and borderline personality disorder."

"I did have PTSD, but I'm no longer having any of the symptoms except anxiety. The borderline personality disorder diagnosis is incorrect. It was given to me by the same physician who overdosed me on amitriptyline."

"Um, okay. Dr. Ersatz will be in shortly." She left the room.

*Shortly* turned out to be forty-five minutes later. A short woman in a long skirt, long-sleeved button-down shirt, and hijab entered the room. She regarded me with cold eyes. "I'm Dr. Ersatz," she said as she sat on her stool. She didn't extend her hand or smile.

"What is your problem with your sleep?" she asked abruptly. Her accent was hard to understand.

"I have a hard time going to sleep at night. My legs won't stop moving. I never had that problem before July of last year when I was given a very high dose of amitriptyline. And I'm exhausted during the day. I wake up every day around six, and I eat breakfast and take care of my dogs. By eight, I'm back in bed because I can't keep my eyes open."

"You drink alcohol. Coffee? Do drugs?"

"Huh? No, I don't drink alcohol. I drink coffee occasionally, maybe a few times a month. I don't do any drugs besides my prescriptions, Zoloft and estradiol."

She gave me a therapist-style stare before rushing through the rest of the interview. "We need some blood and a sleep study. Your restless legs are probably due to iron." She stood up and started to walk from the room. I paused and tried to figure out if I was supposed to stay or go. She made a choppy gesture with her hand. "Come on. My girls will take your blood and check you out."

*My girls?*

I followed Dr. Ersatz into an adjacent room. She gave me no instructions, just turned around and left. I sat in the phlebotomy chair.

After a few minutes, Puffy entered the room. Up close. I could see that her eyes were bloodshot. She too wore a badge that revealed a name but not a position. I wondered if Dr. Ersatz was going for cheap medical assistants instead of nurses. Puffy wore a zip-up hoodie over her scrub top. The hoodie had a bleach stain on the back and was covered in animal hair. I hoped it wasn't cat hair. Cat dander made my chest tight and caused the skin on my hands to swell until the skin split open.

Maybe I should leave and have my labs done elsewhere. But Dr. Ersatz hadn't told me what she was ordering. I guessed she was ordering iron based on her comment, but I wasn't sure if that was all she wanted. Puffy put a tourniquet on my arm and attached a vial to the syringe. She told me to make a fist and took aim. After she'd pulled the needle from my arm, I'd grabbed a cotton ball from the counter and jumped from the chair.

I was still seeing Grace, mostly because I'd gotten into the habit of seeing her. Once I get into a habit, it's hard to break. She was still on her "You need to have more fun!" kick. Like a big idiot, I deferred to her authority. Andrew bought us tickets to see the classical guitarists Rodrigo y Gabriela. I'd loved concerts as a teen, so I'd thought it was a risk worth taking. I knew my relationship to sound was different now, so I took earplugs.

"Are you okay?" I watched Andrew's mouth as he asked the question. I wasn't sure how to answer. I wasn't okay. I couldn't think and my body was in a panic, but still I nodded. He'd spent a lot of money on this rare night out. I didn't want to turn around and leave.

As we walked back to the car after the concert, I realized that when I tried to speak, I couldn't. My words were now jagged and nonsensical. When we got home, I pulled my Royals blanket over my head and slept.

I opened my eyes. Sunlight was diving through the window. I got up to go to the bathroom. Andrew sat in the office drinking coffee. He called out to me as I passed by the office door. I have no idea what he said, but his voice cut through my head like a chainsaw. I screamed, ran into the quilt room, and pulled the door closed behind me. It felt like the insides of my ears were being stabbed with a spike. Andrew followed me.

"What're you doing?" he shouted.

"Oh my God, oh my God," was all I could say as I teared up.

"Twilah, what is your problem?"

"Stop, stop," I screamed. Tears flowed. I tried to push past Andrew into the bedroom. I had to get away from his voice.

"What the fuck?" he yelled.

I shut and locked the bedroom door behind me. I crammed plugs into my ears. I sat in bed and tried to focus on my breathing.

Andrew was banging on the door. "What are you doing?"

"Shut up!" I yelled. I couldn't think. I couldn't find nice words. Pain pulsed through my head. I pulled a pillow over it and continued to cry. After Andrew gave up on his banging, I unlocked the door.

"What is the matter with you?" he barked.

"Please stop. It hurts."

He lowered his voice. "What hurts?"

"Your voice. The birds outside. The lawn mower outside. Everything." I wiped my tears with my hand and pulled my husky onto my lap.

"Do you see Grace soon?"

"Yes."

"Good. I'm coming to see her with you. This is out of control." He turned and walked from the room.

~

As always, the first thing I did upon entering Grace's waiting area was turn the radio off. I sat and scrolled through my phone. Andrew sat next to me and did the same. We hadn't spoken during the drive.

Grace opened the door to her office. "Come in," she said with a smile. "So, what's going on?" she asked after a pause.

Andrew spoke first. "She's yelling and screaming at me for talking to her now. This is out of control."

Grace fixed her gaze on me. "What happened?"

"It's hurting me. He keeps talking to me, and it hurts. I tried to run away, but he just raised his voice louder."

"Sound hurts?" she echoed.

"Yes! It hurts! This hurts now, this talking. It's killing me." The tears had started up again.

"But you're yelling at your husband because of it?"

"I was trying to get away."

"She was screaming and yelling at me," Andrew repeated.

"Because it hurt! It hurts!"

"You still have to pay attention to your behavior," Grace scolded.

Andrew pounced. "Yes, you can't run screaming from me and expect me to understand what's happening."

"Oh my fucking God," I shot back. "If I'd slapped you on your incision after your thoracotomy, do you think you would've been able to calmly ask me to stop? It fucking hurts. I was reacting to *fucking pain!*"

"Even if you think it hurts, you have to pay attention to your behavior," declared Grace.

If I *thought* it hurt? How much thinking did *she* do about pain?

"What else is going on?" she asked. I guessed the discussion was over. *How do therapists decide when a topic is closed?*

"He keeps calling me during the day. I can't handle it anymore," I complained.

"What do you mean?" asked Grace.

"I try to do things while I'm at home. Meditate or whatever, and he calls and interrupts me. He's always done it, and I can't handle it anymore."

Grace stared at me for a bit before speaking. "He cares about you. I don't see a problem with him checking on you."

"I can't handle being interrupted."

"I don't understand. He cares about you," she stated again. She turned her gaze to Andrew. "You call because you care, right?"

"Yes. But fine. If she's going to make it such a big deal, I'll never call again." He turned his reddened face to me. "I won't call ever anymore then. Ever. I'll never do it, okay. Never!"

"Fuck you! You always have to make me seem like the asshole. Whenever I ask you to respect my need to concentrate, you turn it into this big always/never, black/white, *I'm* being unreasonable. Fuck you. I'm done. I can't handle being interrupted. I can't. Okay. I can't focus."

My hands shook with rage. I turned to Grace. "He's never respected what I do in the daytime. Never. He's always had to interrupt me. He called Tuesday, and I said stop calling me. He said okay. Then he called Thursday. I said, 'Don't fucking call me.' So, he called from his Saturday job. I'm *done!*" I shouted.

Grace stared at me. "I don't understand what you're saying," she finally said. "What do you want to hear?"

"I'm saying I've been asking him for years to not call me during the day, and he still fucking does." I buried my face in my hands. "And every fucking time he says he'll stop, he makes it this big dramatic production. 'Oh, I'll never, ever, ever do that again,' and then he does it two days later. Fuck this, I'm done!"

"See, Grace? This is out of control. She flies into a rage over everything. She can't stand any sound at all. The cicadas outside make her cry. She flips out over everything little thing. Last night, she threw her dinner plate against the wall when she saw that her fork didn't match her spoon. She's obsessed with the silverware now. She'll only eat with one set. She can't do anything around the house anymore. It's like she's lost all her skills. I'm constantly worried because she gets confused, goes off wandering, and gets lost. Then I have to drive around until I find her. But then she blows up at me if I call to check on her. She still can't speak at all half the time, and she gets frustrated and smacks her head with her fist when she can't communicate. I can't handle this anymore, Grace. I'm at the end of my rope here," pleaded Andrew.

"Fuck this. Fuck all of you! I'm done!" I screamed.

"What do you mean 'done'?" asked Grace. "What do you want him to say? What do you want to hear?"

*What the fuck does she think* done *means?* And I didn't *want to hear* anything. I wanted my relationship with my husband back. I wanted peace. I wanted quiet. I wanted my brain back. The conversation had become incoherent. I no longer tried to speak. It was clear that neither Grace nor Andrew were going to be receptive to the truth as I was so clearly stating it. I cried into my hands. Fuck them both. Thirty fruitless minutes later, Grace opened the door for us to exit. I reached into my purse and realized I'd forgotten my planner.

"Just call me for another appointment," she said.

"I'm having a really hard time using the phone. I can't hear—" I'd been telling her that for weeks.

"Call me," she repeated before closing the door.

Fuck them all. If I had to remove myself from the company of all of them in order to survive, I would. I'd ditch therapy, ditch the doctors, ditch my husband if I had to. Something had happened to my brain, and it was far more complex than mental illness.

I only saw Grace a couple of more times. When I spoke of my concerns about the rage that accompanied my constant anxiety—how before my brain changed I'd been able to meditate my anger and anxiety away much of the time—she'd simply repeat, "We can't all be Buddhist monks."

Then she'd stare at me. She crossed the final line when I complained about the dirty looks I got from medical receptionists now that I had a Medicare card.

"You *think* they're looking at you differently?" she'd volleyed back.

Thankfully, Andrew and I had patched things up. He'd stepped in and defended me. "Grace, I've worked in health care my entire life since leaving the Air Force. And before the Air Force, I was an EMT on an ambulance. What she's saying is real. I've seen it happen more times than I can count. There's pervasive discrimination in health care culture against people with invisible disabilities."

Her eyes widened. "But why? And what does that have to do with your insurance? Why do they care what insurance you have?"

The sound and stimulations of the day had broken down my ability to speak clearly. "Because they see s-s-someone who looks young and able-bodied. The M-Medicare card tells them that I'm on Social Security Disability. So, they think I'm a lazy sc-sc-scammer."

"I don't understand. I just don't understand. I know you're not lazy. Why do they care about your Medicare?" she repeated the question several times.

Her perspective was simply too privileged to allow her to be of help. She had great insight into the egocentric practice of medicine but none into the day-to-day facts of discrimination against people with disabilities or people of color. She would've never believed me about the Medicare if Andrew hadn't been there to back me up.

Dr. Iyilik had moved from his office with Dr. Thueban to another location. The front office staff at this facility liked to play loud classic rock and country music. Dr. Iyilik knew that sound caused me confusion, and he'd asked the receptionists to turn the music off in advance of my appointments. After his mandate, the women at the front desk had started to glare at me each time I came in.

I never went back. I canceled my next appointment and weaned myself off Zoloft.

# CHAPTER TWENTY-SEVEN

THE RESULTS OF the DaTScan arrived in the mail.

> Normal uptake in the right caudate head. Normal uptake in the left caudate head. Minimally decreased uptake in the right putamen. Normal uptake in the left putamen.
> Impression:
> Minimally decreased uptake in the right putamen, which may represent early Parkinsonism, though normal variant cannot be excluded. If there is persistent clinical concern, examination could be repeated in one year.

That was outside the scope of what Dr. Google and I could understand. I'd have to talk to Dr. Wise to find out what it meant.

Enclosed with the report was a sheet that listed several drugs that the DaTScan manufacturer, GE, had reported to have the potential to interfere with the test results. Sertraline, the generic name for Zoloft, was on the list. And I was still on sertraline. The list went on to name citalopram, fluoxetine, paroxetine, venlafaxine, duloxetine, escitalopram, imipramine, clomipramine, pimozide, and ziprasidone. The decongestants pseudoephedrine and xylometazoline were included as well.

I wondered whether anyone else found it troublesome that medications could cause physical changes that mimicked neurodegenerative conditions in imaging studies. I also wondered if these drugs' ability to mimic neurodegenerative conditions that accompany organic movement disorders meant the drugs could act on the same receptors as the conditions themselves, and in a detrimental fashion.

*Those sound like good questions.*

Yeah, I thought so. Too bad finding someone to discuss them with seemed impossible.

---

My Subaru's engine roared like a jet each time the transmission changed gears. The click of my turn signal sounded like the whap of hollow wood against a wall. The sirens on a passing ambulance prompted tears.

It was September 2015, time for my annual eye exam. I had an eye doctor I really liked, Dr. Able, but she'd moved her office out to the hinterlands of Missouri. I still had a problem with getting lost while driving—though not as often. I read some reviews and decided to try a new eye doctor with an office less than a mile from my home. I figured I'd somehow find my way there and back.

I listened to white noise through my earbuds as I filled out a new-patient history form. In the medical history section, I scribbled that I had an unknown neurological condition.

A woman who looked like she belonged in high school retrieved me from the waiting room. I was surprised when she started to perform the exam. My surprise turned to dismay when she started to test my peripheral vision. Dr. Able's office had always had me look into a device that flashed grey-lined circles within the boundaries of a larger circle. This woman stood in front of me and waved her hands while repeating, "Can you see this? Can you see this?"

I shook my head. The test wasn't objective, the results weren't systematically quantifiable, and the test conditions couldn't be duplicated.

But I didn't want a fight, so I did my best to follow her directions.

"I need you to hold your eyes still, please," she repeated several times. Since late 2014, my eyes had begun to jerk and dance in a way they'd never done.

A second woman in a white lab coat entered the room. She introduced herself, but I couldn't understand her name.

"Stop moving your eyes!" she barked.

"I'm dooing m-m-my best." The effort it took to understand their speech and sounds in the office had gotten to me. "They won't s-s-stop mooving."

"Okay, take out your contacts," she instructed. The doctor, who was now a white blob, left the room and came back with new lenses. "Try these on," she instructed before turning and leaving again. I got up from the exam chair and found my way to the counter, where I thought Dr. Bitchy Blob had set the lenses. I pressed them onto my eyes but still couldn't see. Blob returned. "How are the contacts?" she asked.

"I still can't see. I d-d-don't know how much the dilation is a factor, but this p-p-prescription doesn't seem right. Everything's blurry. I can't focus at all."

She puffed out a loud breath. "Did you even put them in the right eyes? I bet you mixed them up!"

I knew I hadn't. I'd paid careful attention when I'd inserted them.

"I'm pretty s-s-sure I got it right, but I'd be h-h-happy to try again while you watch."

Blob let out a puff of air and walked briskly from the room again. A couple of minutes later, she entered with more contacts. She stood almost on top of me while I inserted them.

"No," I said. "I still can't see. I can't focus. This isn't the right prescription."

"Yes, it is!" she shouted.

"I put on my form that I have a neurological condition. I'm

doing the best I c-c-can. I'd like a pair of contacts in my o-o-original prescription, and I'd like to leave now."

Bitchy Blob spun around and left the room again. After a brief moment, she returned. She slapped down more contacts on the counter. I put them in my eyes. "Y-y-yeah. These are better, but I still can't f-focus."

"I don't know what to tell you. The dilation wouldn't do that, and your prescription is correct. Check out down the hall and to your right," she said before leaving the room.

The following week, Andrew took me to see my old optometrist, Dr. Able. At Andrew's request, the receptionist turned off the overhead music. My thoughts remained clear. I told Dr. Able about my visit to Dr. Blob.

"I'm sorry that happened," Dr. Able replied. "Lots of the larger clinics have techs do the majority of the exam. That's the first problem. Then there are a few patients whose behind-the-mask prescription turns out to be different from the prescription they need in real life. It's uncommon, but not unheard of. If that doctor hasn't been in practice long, she might not have known that."

As Dr. Able walked me through the exam, she didn't scold me for my inability to hold my dancing eyes still.

"I haven't seen anything like this. Is there a treatment or cure for these neurological events you're experiencing?" she asked.

"Not that I know of. But I'm not really sure that what's happened to me has been very well understood by the neurologists I've seen."

"Well, don't give up," she encouraged. "It was good seeing you again. Thanks for coming all the way up here. Let me know if there are any problems with the contacts or if you have any other concerns."

❧

I folded my Royals blanket and set it in the bottom of my duffel bag. I was packing for my sleep study. I didn't give a damn about baseball, but it was the perfect weight. I brought my perfectly firm pillow, which was encased in fabric of precisely the right texture.

And, of course, I wore earplugs. These sensitivities were new. Before 2014, I would've been able to sleep with whatever had been provided.

Dr. Ersatz entered the exam room forty-five minutes after my scheduled appointment time. I shifted my eyes to her pretty red plaid hijab and smiled. As I opened my mouth to compliment her headscarf, she aimed her cold eyes at me and spoke. I watched the pleasant words I'd formed in my mind dissolve.

"Your study says you have sleep apnea," she declared. She delivered the words with the tone of a judge proclaiming me guilty of murder. "You need to have another sleep study to set the pressure on the CPAP machine." She continued launching words at me, but I couldn't follow her clipped, accented speech.

I knew my expression had become blank. Dr. Ersatz's eyes became colder in response. "That's it," she declared as she stood. "We need your vitamin D and iron levels again. Both were low last time."

"What were they?" I asked.

She sighed and flipped through some papers in her lap. She read off a few numbers. I didn't understand her, but I noticed she hadn't stated units of measurement. I wondered if she knew the units of measurement.

"Can I have a copy of my sleep study and my lab results please?"

Her brows were angry dark rivets pushing down toward her nose. Her forehead was creased. "It's all in the portal," she spat as she waved me through the door and back into the small phlebotomy area.

"I've tried logging into the portal, and I can't get in. How can I get in?" I asked.

"Ask the girls," she said as she walked from the room.

The appointment had taken less than five minutes after my forty-five-minute wait. I took a seat in the phlebotomy chair and waited some more. I wondered if I'd get Puffy the Pet Hair Lady again. A different young woman came in. She put a tourniquet around my arm and offered me a ball.

"Squeeze this," she instructed.

I looked at the stained, pockmarked foam ball she held, and fear rippled through me. I didn't want to touch it. But I also didn't want an argument, so I squeezed the filthy thing.

"How do I log into the portal?"

After some discussion among the "girls," I was given a set of directions that I scribbled in my notebook.

A few days later, I logged into the portal. After clicking around for several minutes, I found my labs and a synopsis of my appointment.

> Assessment and Plan
> The following list includes any diagnoses that were discussed at your visit:
> Sleep apnea
> Sleep apnea: care instructions
> Sleep study referral: titration study
> Sleep paralysis
> REM sleep behavior disorder
> Fatigue
> Vitamin D deficiency

I didn't remember her mentioning sleep paralysis or REM sleep behavior disorder. I continued to scroll. My medication list hadn't been updated, even though I'd given an updated list to her assistant. My primary care provider's information was wrong too. I shook my head, stretched, and got up to check the mail. In it was an error-riddled bill from Dr. Ersatz's office.

I sent a message through the portal and requested a correction to my bill. My brain was grinding to a halt. My thoughts were beginning to disconnect. I gathered up my dogs and slept.

෴

I'd gone back to my Googling. Ha-ha! No, seriously, I'd done some more reading online, and I'd found there's a word for abnormal sensitivity to everyday sound: *hyperacusis*.

"This started when I was having ECT treatments," I referred

to my notes as I explained the timeline to the audiologist. "I had a hormone-based mood disorder called premenstrual dysphoric disorder, but it took forever to find a doctor who took the hormone-based part seriously. Because of that, it got treated for years as regular depression that was refractory to treatment. So, I got desperate and tried ECT. That's when I started hearing the music that wasn't there."

"What did the music sound like?" Dr. Affable asked. "Was it music you recognized?"

"Well, I say music, but it wasn't music per se. It was a series of tones that sounded melodic. I guess that's a better way to describe it."

She looked up from her notepad. "Do you still hear this music?"

"No, it's gone."

"What about ringing in your ears. Do you have that?"

"Yes. After the music went away, I just heard this screaming sound in my ears instead. I wouldn't say *ringing* necessarily. It's more like a high-pitched squeal. It's only in my left ear now."

Affable led me to a small room where she inserted a small wired device into my right ear.

"You'll hear some clicks. You don't need to do anything but sit there."

I nodded my understanding.

A few minutes into the test, she asked, "How are you doing?"

"I'm okay. The clicks hurt, but I'm alright."

"Okay, then we're done."

I wouldn't learn until months later that she'd terminated the test prematurely based on my response to her question.

Next, I was taken to a soundproof booth. I raised my hand each time I heard a tone sound through the headphones Dr. Affable had placed on my head.

"Your hearing is normal," Dr. Affable said as she held open the door of the booth. I'd been told the same thing in college.

A few days later, I returned for more tests. Another audiologist placed a device that looked like a giant viewfinder on my face. She told me to look at a dot and hold my eyes still. My eyes still flitted and danced, but not as intensely as they'd done during my eye exams. The audiologist didn't reproach me for my inability to hold them still.

I went back for my results the following week. "Hi, I'm Dr. Fluké," said the smiling blonde as she extended her hand. I stood and shook it like I'd learned to do in the insurance world, then I returned to my seat.

"This is interesting. As you know, your hearing test was normal. You don't have any vestibular problems. But you clearly have severe hyperacusis. We didn't test your hearing for higher than normal frequencies because there's no normative data to compare the results to. But there is some question as to whether you may be hearing higher frequencies than most people."

She continued, "It's really interesting that you experienced musical tinnitus. That's the rarest form. Do you still have it?"

Musical—*T-I-N*—I started to spell what sounded like an unfamiliar word—*Oh, tinnitus*, I realized. She was pronouncing it differently than I would have expected. "Oh, the music I heard that wasn't there?" I asked after the long pause I'd taken to sort out her meaning.

Dr. Fluké nodded.

"No, it's gone now."

"Weren't you exposed to some drugs that have the potential to damage the auditory system? Do you have a list of the medications that you took?" she asked.

"Not on me, but I can print one for you."

"When did you start having these other symptoms?"

"Um, I can't remember all the dates, but I have a timeline at home. I can get it you."

"Okay, that's fine. How often do you wear earplugs?"

"Um, every day."

"How often throughout the day?"

"At least 90 percent of the time." I thought hard. That may have been an underestimate. I opened my mouth to correct myself, but she'd started speaking again.

"We'll start by trying to get you to reduce that. You see, the more you block out sound, the harder your ears try to hear, which makes the hyperacusis worse in the long run."

I nodded. That seemed possible, but I'd made a note to look into the science behind her statement.

"What kind of earplugs so you wear?"

I visualized them. "I have some foam ones, and then I also have this other kind made of, I don't know, waxy stuff that's custom molded. I wear those in the shower. I also listen to white noise with my Bose to block out sound when I have to go out."

"We can start by transitioning you to blah-blah-blah plugs. They let in more sound. And the data says it's better to listen to pink noise than to white. Do you have pink noise?" She'd mentioned a brand of earplugs, but I couldn't understand what she'd said. It was an odd word I'd never heard before, so I couldn't spell it.

". . . or blah-blah-blah pink noise generator."

I realized I'd missed much of what she'd been saying.

"Can you write that down, please? I have pink noise on my app. I'll start using that."

"Sure!" Dr. Fluké agreed. "It's all about restoring your ability to tolerate sound—getting you to the point where you don't get anxious in anticipation of a noisy environment, getting past that fear."

I opened my mouth to correct her, but she'd moved on. Sound didn't make me anxious. It made me confused.

"What did Dr. Wise say about all of this?" she asked.

"He thinks this is a medication reaction that was made possible by extended exposure to psych meds, especially Abilify," I explained.

She flipped through my chart. "Okay. It's good that you're seeing him. He's a great investigator. Oh, I see you went to see a doctor at Wash U too! That's where I went to school. Blah-blah-blah-blah—"

When she spoke the name of the school, I struggled to sort through her words. Letters appeared and dissolved in my mind. *O-A-U-S-H, no. W-A-W-A, no. A-H-C-H-O-O, no. Oh! W-A-S-H-U!* By the time I figured it out, she'd moved on again. I'd missed everything she'd said in the last couple of minutes while puzzling over that name.

I looked up and realized that Fluké had stood and was extending her hand again. I rose from my seat and shook it. I liked how she'd explained her thought process. She was wrong about the anxiety part, but I could clear that up. I just had to figure out how to follow up with her at a cost of $175 per visit that wasn't covered by insurance.

A few days later, I dropped off a letter.

*September 28, 2015*
*Dear Dr. Fluké,*

*Thank you for the appointment to discuss and treat my hyperacusis. I'm sorry I was not able to better explain the sequence of events leading to my seeking treatment at your office at the time I was seen. I hope that between this letter and the records you get from Dr. Wise, the sequence of events leading up to my appointment will become clearer.*

*I do want to make very clear that my reaction to noise is not fear based. I do not have a psychological or physiological reaction in anticipation of sound. I experience confusion in correlation with loud or prolonged sound exposure, and when the exposure is reduced, my cognition is restored. I experience fear in response to confusion, not vice versa. I become afraid when it becomes evident that my confusion is interfering with my cognition and decision-making skills.*

*I've attempted many times over the course of the past year to become relaxed when I experience confusion or to "think myself out of it," but those efforts have been unsuccessful. I'm an experienced meditator and I can often meditate/think/concentrate myself out of anxious states, but not out of confused states. Once I experience profound confusion, the only antidotes I've found are sleep and the elimination of sound.*

*I make this point because based on the conversation we had at my appointment, it sounded as if you believe I have an aversion to sound that is somewhat akin to anxiety. That's not what's happening. I avoid sounds in order to avoid a loss of cognitive functioning, not to avoid a mood or feeling.*

*I'm sorry I was unable to communicate my experiences more clearly at the time of my appointment. Please review this information and any information you get from Dr. Wise, so that an appropriate course of treatment can be determined for my condition. I think that between the education and experience that you two share, it's possible that a solution to my challenges can be found. Please feel free to bill me for any time associated with the review of this letter.*

*Thank you for your time and consideration.*

*Sincerely,*
*Twilah Hiari*
*Encl: Timeline of onset of symptoms and pharmaceutical history*

~❧~

When I finally got a copy of Dr. Fluké's diagnosis and treatment notes, I saw that she'd characterized my experience as "an unusual presentation of hyperacusis."

**You were getting somewhere in terms of receiving an accurate diagnosis.**

Almost. I also think Dr. Fluké thought I was crazy. She put this in her report too: "She has been followed extensively, and has been diagnosed with general anxiety and depression, PMDD, conversion disorder, and most recently, functional movement disorder."

But she was nice to my face, and that was a really welcome change.

# CHAPTER TWENTY-EIGHT

"HI, MY NAME is Dr. Bland," said the thin brunette. "I'll be administering your neuropsychiatric assessment."

Based on the grey streaks in her hair and the wrinkles near her mouth, I guessed she was in her fifties. We sat down at a small round table.

I offered Dr. Bland copies of my college transcript and LSAT scores. I suspected Dr. Crow and Dr. Jape had refused to believe my cognition had changed partly because they'd had no evidence of how incredibly well I'd been able to think before my injury.

Dr. Bland interviewed me about my life much like Dr. Anjān had. I offered as succinct a synopsis of my childhood as I could in response to her questions.

"You weren't sexually assaulted, were you?" Dr. Bland interjected as I tried to explain how I hadn't had a stable place to live as a teen.

"Yeah, I was."

"Ya ever get any help for that?" She glanced up from her legal pad as she spoke. Her brows were pinched in a way that seemed vaguely disapproving.

*Bitch, we do not have time to go into my history with idiot therapists who denied the possibility that I could have encountered trauma,* I thought, before taking a breath and offering a more tempered response. "I think I worked on that with my last therapist."

Dr. Bland lowered her head and scribbled on her legal pad. I suppressed the temptation to scratch onto my thigh the letters of the words she spoke. I pressed my hands flat into my lap to keep my fingers still. I didn't want her to mischaracterize what I now know is self-stimulatory behavior, what we call stimming, as common anxiety and tell me my problems were psychogenic.

"Make sure you get a good night's sleep before the test. The testing will last a few hours, so you should bring a snacky-wacky," she concluded with a slight upward turn of her lips.

I paused. *Snacky-wacky? Had I heard her right?* Andrew's somewhat disgusted expression told me that I had. I took a breath and decided to ignore her attempt to infantilize me. Since my cognition and behavior had changed, most everyone treated me like a child.

Two weeks later, I was back. Midway through the tests, Bland turned on a fan. As the noise reached my ears, my brain had begun to struggle. But I didn't protest. I knew the enormous effort it would take to create words to ask her to turn off the fan, and then the processing of her response to my request would be even more disruptive than the sound of the fan itself. I felt my brain slowing and exhaustion setting in.

Weeks later, we returned for the results.

"I'll give you a copy of the full report when it's ready, but right now I want to discuss areas on the test where your scores varied significantly from what would have been expected based on your prior metrics of performance—your college GPA and your LSAT scores," she started. She rattled off an explanation, but I couldn't keep up with her words.

I glanced at her legal pad and saw that she'd written the word *Caucasian* across the top. After she stopped talking, I spoke.

"I'm not Caucasian," I said. "Nobody asked me about my ethnic background."

That had sent her into a quick tempo explanation of the role of race in IQ testing. I couldn't follow that any better than I'd been able to follow her explanation of my test results. I gained more insight when a copy of her report arrived in the mail.

> Simple visual attention and scanning is above average, although performance on the Visual Working Memory Index of the Wechsler Memory Scale-IV is 21 percentile and lower than predicted. Performance is low average for attending to dots across pages and identifying symbol stands in serial order.
>
> With regard to visual spatial skills . . . below average in copying a design, in that her score is 31/36. Minor errors are noted in integrating details and use of space.
>
> Visual Memory Index is 37 percentile. Immediate recall of designs and location and immediate recall and reproduction of figures is high average, but delayed recall of both are below average.
>
> Delayed Memory Index is predicted to be a standard score of 109 and it is 92, which is lower than expected.
>
> Verbal abstraction reasoning and concept formation is above average, through rapid semantic fluency is low average to average.
>
> Neuropsychological Implications: Ms. Hiari presents as a woman well above average in native intellectual ability. This is consistent with LSAT score (88th percentile). The profile reveals difficulty on some tasks of auditory and visual attention, delayed recall, and tasks of executive functions. Correlation with medical tests is advised. It is likely the profile reflects the combined impact of sensory

motor changes, fatigue, and history of amitriptyline use. Hyperacusis and fatigue are likely interrelated and mutually exacerbating.

Diagnosis:
The test profile yields evidence of DSMV Axis III referral diagnoses of Other Amnesia/Memory Loss and Axis I diagnosis of Cognitive DO/Other Signs and Symptoms with Cognitive Functions and Awareness.

*⁓&*

*Dr. Bland's testing finally quantified the cognitive problems you'd been reporting for over a year?*

Yeah, yeah it did. But it still understated them. My memory hadn't been average before the brain changes—it had been phenomenal. When I'd been at Indemnity National, I'd had between eighty and 120 claim files at any given time, and I'd been able to correlate the last six digits of each sixteen-digit claim number with the claimant's name, the facts of the accident, and the year, make, and model of the vehicle. I don't know anybody else in the office who could do that. But there was no way to prove how amazing my memory had been before 2014.

# CHAPTER TWENTY-NINE

"I'VE REVIEWED YOUR test results," Dr. Wise said. "The DaTScan probably reflected the effect of the Zoloft, so I don't think those findings are clinically significant. Are you still taking Zoloft?"

"No. I stopped it a while ago, right after I learned I can't metabolize it. I started taking probiotics, and my anxiety started getting better, so I weaned myself off the Zoloft."

"Good. Your neuropsych results were encouraging. You performed really well in some areas, so I think with time you can expect your memory and other weaker areas to improve." He continued, "How's your sleep? I haven't gotten a report from Dr. Ersatz yet."

"I'm still exhausted. I can't get through the day without at least a couple of naps. And I have terrible insomnia at night—and nightmares, and restless legs. She said I have sleep apnea, but I really didn't like the way she communicated. I'm going to get a second opinion."

"That sounds like a good idea."

I knew there was a bigger answer to why my brain changes had happened.

I had to talk to Burt. He'd cleared up many of my mother's other lies. She'd always insisted that he'd been a deadbeat after their divorce. She'd said she'd lost the home I'd lived in as a child due to a clause in the divorce that made her surrender it if she married again. He'd produced receipts for the child support he'd paid as well as for the payments he'd sent for the mortgage on the house. There'd been no clause about the house in the divorce paperwork. She'd squandered all the money Burt sent, and the bank had foreclosed on our home.

I plugged in my Bose. "Hi, hon." I strained to hear Burt's soft voice. "Sorry it took me awhile to call you back. I've been drivin' over the road again."

"Oh wow," I said. "I'm glad you're healthy enough to do that." I knew Department of Transportation physicals were rigorous, and he was a triple bypass survivor.

"Well, we need the money," he replied. I guessed that by "we," he meant him, Patricia, and Patricia's disabled adult son. "How've you been, hon?"

"Um, I've been kinda sick. That's why I'm calling. I have some questions about my health when I was younger."

I heard him exhale. "Wanna meet somewhere and get somethin' ta eat?"

"I'd like to, but I can't stand sound anymore. I can't eat out because it's too loud. You can come over here."

"Well, we'll see. What did you wanna know?"

"I remember Mom always talking about how I was sick when I was a baby. Is this true? Was I really sick?"

"Yeahhhh." He pulled on the word. "You was allergic to anything and everything. You was a picky eater too. Real picky. Your mom got you set up with some doctor, down off I-70 and Eighteenth Street—down thataways. I took you to that doctor, and he gave ya shots in both your legs, between your thigh and knee, right around ther."

My eyes were clamped shut with concentration. I wrote down what he told me, struggling to make block letters I could read later.

"How old was I? What were the shots for?"

"You woulda been young. You'd just started to walk. I took you every week for these shots. The doctor said it was for an immune somethin' or other. You grew outta the shots round the time you started school."

"Do you remember me actually being sick or just the shots?"

"Well, I was on the road a lot. I know you had pneumonia real bad when you was a little baby. You was always sick with somethin'. Your mom took care of most of the doctors' visits and stuff though. I was driving."

"But you took me for these shots."

"Yeah," he said without further explanation.

Burt and I talked for over an hour. When the conversation ended, I knew more about myself, my brothers, Burt, and my mother than I'd ever known. The effort to understand his voice had left me exhausted. I set my notes aside and went to sleep.

***

Andrew helped me figure out which buzzer corresponded to which apartment in the high-rise. The chart was too confusing for me to sort out. I pressed the button he pointed out, and the door clicked open. We rode the elevator to the sixth floor.

"Hi, hon," Mom said as she pulled me to her chest. Andrew hung back behind me.

"Hi, Mom. Thanks for having us over."

"Well, it's good having my kids in my life again. I hope this is gonna be a nice visit again. I hope you're not coming at me." Her blue eyes were fearful.

"Mom, if you promise not to lie to me anymore, I won't come at you again. I need information, okay—true, legitimate information. If you lie, I'll just turn around and leave. You won't have to worry about me coming *at* you again. I'll leave, and you'll never see me again. Okay?"

"I'm sorry, hon, but everything you wanna blame me for is in the past. The past is the past. Let it go. I won't lie. I promise you.

God's truth. I want my kids back in my life." Her raspy voice caught on her words.

"I didn't come here to blame you for anything." I told my mind to let my rising anger dissipate.

"Well then, how have you been, baby girl?"

I smiled. Did my mother actually care about me now? "I've been sick, Mom. I had this hormone-based mood disorder that made me depressed—"

"There ya go! You're not like me. I've always been strong. You've always been weak!" She was beyond her fear now. She flashed a big smile.

I clenched my jaw and dug my fingernails into my palms. I would not let her get to me. "I came here to ask you about some things that have to do with my sickness—my weakness, I guess. I remember you always told me I was sick as a baby. I need to know about that."

Her eyes lit up, and her wrinkles seemed to flatten. Her smile widened even more, and I saw that she only had a few teeth left. "Oh yes. Yes, you were. You were almost like the boy in the bubble! You had an immune deficiency. They had to give you blah-blah-blah-blah injections." The pride in her voice was unmistakable.

"Now I know what you're thinking," she went on. "It isn't that disease the blacks get. I had you tested for that black disease as soon as you were born. You know their diseases are different than ours."

"Um, do you mean sickle cell anemia?" I asked.

"Yeah, that. You don't have that."

"When did I first get sick?" I steered her back.

"You were always sick. You had pneumonia four times before you were a year old. You had all kinds of breathing problems and infections and this and that. You were allergic to everything. I took you to this allergy specialist, out there in Johnson County. He did some tests and said you were allergic to horses and snow! I said *'What? She's never been around horses.'* But that's what the doctor said—horses and snow!"

I looked at Andrew. The skepticism in his face was clear. I raised a brow at him.

"Did the doctor tell you that Twilah was allergic to ordinary things too, or just horses and snow?" he redirected her.

"What, hon? Oh yeah. He said mold and I think tomatoes." Her voice had lost its enthusiasm. This was too mundane to hold her interest. There was no exoticism in mold and tomatoes. "You had asthma too!"

"I remember the asthma," I said. *No surprise with her smoking all the time*, I thought. "But what about the tomato allergy? How did I do with other foods?"

"You were such a picky eater! The pickiest. Glen and Jeffrey would eat everything. Not you. You were so picky! Picky Mickey! That's why you were such a Skinny Minnie!" she hooted. "You were tiny. Sometimes you didn't grow at all! You wore the same-sized clothes for two years. I didn't have to buy you any new outfits from the time you were three to the time you were five! Saved me some money!"

I wanted to take a deep breath to center myself, but my lungs urged me not to inhale too deeply in the smoke-filled hovel. I settled for rubbing my hands on my jeans and rocking gently in my seat.

"Tell me about these injections I had."

"They were blah-blah-blah injections. They gave 'em to ya right in your thighs. It just broke my heart, baby girl! You'd just started to walk, and those shots sent you right back to crawling. Broke your mama's heart!" she howled. I glanced up at a reproduction of a wolf on the wall. The grey animal had its head thrown back. I imagined it sounded a lot like my mother. "You're lucky they didn't put you in the bubble, like in the movie! They talked about it. You were almost the girl in the bubble!"

I had no idea what bubble or movie she was talking about, but I knew I had to redirect her before she tried to explain. My ears had been peppered with so many television and movie plot synopses while growing up that my brain could still feel the numbness. Television was the highest authority in my mother's life. It resided in a realm of holiness beyond God and time.

"Mom, how long did I have these injections? Over what period of time?"

"Well, they stopped them before you started kindergarten, so before 1980. They said to hold off on your shots too, so you didn't have any of those until right before kindergarten either. You didn't have a single one. But the school required 'em. So, they gave 'em to you all at once, right before school, instead of on the schedule like your brothers had."

"They gave her *all* her vaccinations at once? What were the names of these doctors?" Andrew sounded alarmed.

"Let's see, your pediatrician was Dr. Hancock. Then there was a Dr. Cox and a Dr. White, I think." She was looking up at the ceiling trying to recollect the names. I scribbled in my notepad.

We sat for a bit longer and permitted Mom to digress and ramble. She lectured us on Tony Stewart's driving performance that year. She called him "Smoke" and acted like he was a close friend.

She segued from that into a monologue about her neighbors. "You don't know what I go through living here in housing, baby girl. My neighbor across the hall, she's a drunk. They've got the drunks and druggers and hardcore mentals in here. This is public housing, baby girl. It's bad. It's not the nice world you all live in."

I absorbed her words. She had no idea where I lived, and she knew nothing about my life over the many years I'd spent away from her. She'd never asked.

Finally, I stood. "Well, thanks, Mom. We've gotta go home and feed our dogs."

I tensed as she pulled me into an embrace and slobbered a wet kiss onto my cheek. "Good seeing you, baby girl. And nice seeing you, Alex." She reached for my husband, and I could see his lips pull back at the corners. He disliked being touched as much as I did. He stepped back and patted her on the shoulder. He avoided her embrace by guiding her gently toward her walker. She smiled, revealing her four remaining teeth, before leaning over to plant another kiss on my cheek.

"I'll tell ya goodbye and I love ya," she sang out as the door closed behind us.

"Love you too, Mom."

"She's a fuckin' loon," declared Andrew minutes later as he started the car.

"I know. I know. But what about the stuff she said? From a medical standpoint? What does it mean?"

"Well, if she's telling the truth about the blah-blah-blah injections, that's somewhat interesting," he started.

"Hold on," I interrupted. "What was she saying? I could never understand that word."

"G-A-M-M-A, G-L-O-B-U-L-I-N," he spelled. "It's a plasma product. They give it to some cancer patients. We worked with it at the oncology lab. It gives an immunocompromised person passive immunity. Like, if a person doesn't have their own immunity, they can get some immunity from the donor. That's passive immunity."

"Could it be true? Me getting these injections? Is that something that happened in the '70s, or is it totally make believe?"

"I'd have to look it up. I was born in 1969, honey. I've only been a clinical scientist since the '90s." He smiled. "But if they did do it back then, I'd be concerned about the potential for contamination. In those days, blood products weren't screened the way they are now."

"And this allergy to snow? And horses?"

"I've never heard of a snow allergy. And I'm not an allergist, but I thought you had to have some degree of exposure to an allergen for it to show on a test. You grew up in the city. Were you ever around horses?"

"No."

I pulled up Google and skimmed articles as he drove. Gamma globulin was an immunoglobulin that came from plasma from a large donor pool. In the 1970s, that pool had largely been prison inmates and inhabitants of impoverished areas of large American cities like Los Angeles.

"Do you think there could be epigenetic repercussions because of exposure to that much foreign biomatter? Like, could it activate dormant genetic potential for disease in my body?"

"Sure is something to think about, isn't it?" Andrew answered.

At that time, I was also exchanging letters with my older half-brother, Glen, who was incarcerated in New York. He'd offered his memories of the weekly injections I'd had to treat my immune deficiency as a baby.

I'd always believed I'd been healthy prior to the onset of the PMDD. I'd based that belief on the fact I hadn't been hospitalized for anything physical as an adult. Now, I saw my health history in a new light.

Hadn't the kidney infection in 2003 been unusual for an otherwise healthy person? What about the cold sores I had throughout the '90s that had always turned into oozing staph infections? The pneumonia in 2000? I seemed to get bronchitis annually. I'd contracted pink eye when no one around me had that infection. And what about the many allergic reactions I'd had over the years? I'd had reactions so severe after exposure to soy and cat hair that the skin around my tattoos had swelled up and started to burn. I hadn't had a new tattoo in more than a decade, but my body seemed to periodically reject the ink.

And there were the strange episodes of chest pain. I ended up in the ER about once a year when that happened. What had looked like relative health now appeared to be relative sickness.

My mother's lies had rendered me unable to tell truth from fiction. I knew she'd have me rely on misinformation even if the consequences of applying that misinformation in my life were disastrous. But this story of my immune deficiency as a child had now been confirmed by Burt and Glen. I had to reevaluate the foundational facts of my life one more time.

---

*Why was your brother incarcerated? It seems like your mother correctly foretold his future, even if she was wrong about yours.*

Huh? Oh. He's in prison for child porn. Here's the crazy thing: When he was in the county jail, before he went to prison, I sent him this scathing letter. I told him that every single image he'd ever viewed or distributed represented abuse and exploitation, sometimes even slavery. I wanted him to know that if he was involved in that shit, it wasn't just some abstract matter of pictures—it was a matter of lives seriously being altered, potentially stolen. Bodies and souls destroyed. I wasn't soft, and I didn't mince words.

But here's where things got confusing: He wrote back and said that none of the images he'd had were of children, and that none had involved sex acts. He told me they'd all been striptease-type images of what he believed were women eighteen and older, and that he'd downloaded them from sites that claimed they were legal. I looked up the statute he was convicted under, and it specifically pertained to images of children under sixteen. I'd think the prosecutor would've had to convince the judge that the images were of people under sixteen to convict him under that law. I would think that if the images were as grey as Glen claims they were, it wouldn't have been possible to convict him.

So, I was puzzled by his response. If he was telling the truth, I don't get how he'd made the mistake he was claiming to have made about thinking he was looking at grown women. Personally, I think anyone under age twenty-five looks about twelve years old, you know what I mean? I see people driving, and I'm like, *My God, I thought you had to be out of elementary school to get a license!* I can't imagine mistaking a sixteen-year-old for an adult. And furthermore, I can't imagine thinking of a young-looking person in a sexual way.

I think there might be something wrong with Glen's brain that makes it so he can't distinguish adults from children. And from what Burt and Mom told me, it sounds like he had PANS when he was four. You know?

**Yes, I've heard of PANS—pediatric acute-onset neuropsychiatric syndrome.**

Yeah. PANS accounts for how both Burt and Mom said he was a normal kid until he got an infection and had a fever of 104 degrees for several days. They said after that, he went berserk. He got violent and crazy. Burt said it was like he was demon possessed. Mom says his eyes even looked red—glowing red. That's when he'd attacked her with a knife.

I think my family has some weird hereditary-susceptibility things going on. Glen was born in 1966. His infection would've been in 1970, so think of the state of medical science back then. I'm not trying to excuse his behavior. He belongs in prison if he had child porn. But if there are other factors involved, it'd be interesting to know the whole story. Maybe we could keep people from turning out like him.

*That's interesting. Why did Andrew look concerned when your mother mentioned vaccines? Did he think they played a role in your autism?*

No. He wondered whether getting all of my childhood vaccines in one visit instead of spread-out over the prior years might have overwhelmed my immune system. That's before he'd thought on it and realized that even if I had gotten all my vaccines at once, the vaccine schedule in 1980 still would've resulted in me getting far fewer vaccines in one day than kids get now.

But it's kind of inevitable we'd get to a point where that question is asked, isn't it? Vaccines and autism—is there a link?

I'd started showing signs of autism well before I was first vaccinated. I confirmed all that with Burt—that I'd had late vaccinations and that I'd had behaviors that would be considered autistic. I had those behaviors before kindergarten.

But let me tell you what else I've figured out. People can and do have adverse neurological reactions to vaccines. I mean, that's indisputable. There are a whole lot of documented vaccine injuries; this isn't some fringe notion. There've been demonstrated relationships between vaccines and acute disseminated encephalomyelitis. Huh? I'll write it down for you, look it up. Some people get other kinds of encephalitis and encephalopathies.

So, do I think kids can have neuropsychiatric injuries because of vaccines? Absolutely. I mean, look at what pharmaceuticals did to my brain. There's no question that some of these pharmaceuticals can cause brain changes to people with certain immunological characteristics. Imagine if I'd been injured when my brain was developing. Imagine how that might've looked. As an adult, my brain had already established pathways of functioning it wanted to revert to. A developing brain might establish completely novel pathways in the face of a toxic injury.

But when kids have vaccine reactions that affect their behavior and cognition, they're experiencing something other than old-school autism. I think what they're having is more like PANS. I call what they have pseudoautism, since it looks like autism but isn't quite the same as congenital autism. It's an event that makes what was once a neurotypical kid share some of the qualities you find in autism, but worse. Autism would be really unique if we found out it's a medical condition that *isn't* affected by environmental factors, especially considering how rapidly it's increasing in prevalence.

You're what, in your sixties? Do you seriously believe there have always been this many autistic people? I don't. I mean, yes, there have always been undiagnosed autistics like me. People of my generation and older people too. But most of us don't look like these young autistics. Old-school autism was hyperrationality, hypersensitivity, and science-mindedness with a big dose of social ineptitude. Yeah, I'm emotional, but my emotions don't *motivate* me in terms of big decisions—reason does. These young autistics aren't rational. They're very emotionally motivated and irrational. They couldn't reason their way out of a paper bag. When they hear something they don't like, they start melting down and calling for censorship. They make their decisions based on feelings, not reason. They're more like neurotypical people with brain damage than people with Asperger's.

It isn't the same condition, or it's a significant exacerbation or mutation of the same condition. These youngsters, these so-called neurodiversity proponents—I call them Stockholm syndrome autistics. They're all injured, but between swallows of ADHD meds, they're shouting from the rooftops that their autism wasn't caused by anything chemical or environmental. The hell it wasn't. Do you remember my therapist Jane? I saw several therapists after her when I was in my twenties, and none of them were remotely understanding of my struggles with communication.

Do you think they would've all been so oblivious to the reason for my communication problems if they'd had tons of autistic clients? One of them had worked in Osawatomie for years and still didn't understand why I couldn't speak when I wanted to. She'd never had a client who couldn't speak in meetings or classrooms. So, I don't want to hear that bullshit about how the autistics were in institutions. They weren't. I remember visiting Glen at one of the big group homes he'd been in; it was what some people would call an institution. There were no feces-smearing, head-banging autistics there—none! And beyond anecdote, look at the numbers. If *every single person* in *every single institution* in the US in the '60s, '70s, and '80s had been autistic, it still wouldn't match the numbers of autistics we see today.

I was the only freak like me at any of the four high schools I went to. I hadn't seen another autistic person since preschool. Now, every school in the nation is filled with autistic kids. We're seeing a complete transformation of our species right before our eyes. Historical neurodiversity, my ass. Let's see what these autistic kids look like at my age, after they've been popping psych meds for twenty-plus years.

But you know what? No matter what the cause of autism, I'll take it. If I had to live my early life over and choose either neurotypical or autistic, I'd stand in the line where they hand out autism. Because I love who I am. I love how I think. You all might have tried to crush that, but you couldn't. I can't think of any other way I could've survived what I've been through. My hyperrationality helped me survive. It gave me the power to look at things logically when neurotypical people would have been blinded by emotions and a craving for belonging and social approval.

It woulda been a never-ending struggle of being dragged down by emotionally based decision-making. My emotions are more satisfied with access to knowledge than relationships with people. If I'd been neurotypical, I would've done more stupid shit to fit in. Because fitting in would've been an option. I might've had the long list of abusive exes, and the house full of kids, the drug habit, and all that other shit that people with childhoods like mine so often end up with.

But those are only strengths in a dysfunctional world that no one should have to live in. In the context of a loving family and society, the solitary aspects of autism aren't as useful. They divide a person from others, rather than uniting them with their community.

And the other thing is, there's a sweet spot—a degree of autism where the balance of the condition is more helpful than hurtful. That's what I had before 2014, and that's what I want back. I love my hyperfocus. I love my analytical thought processes. But I hate getting disoriented and confused. I hate my inability to tolerate sound. I hate becoming completely nonverbal. There's a difference between a congenital brain difference and an iatrogenic injury. I didn't consent to this state. No one told me this could happen.

# CHAPTER THIRTY

NOVEMBER 2015. I still couldn't drive most of the time. I'd either get lost or get so fixated on the motion around me that I'd have to pull over, park, and wait for my brain to clear. Andrew took me to my appointment with my new sleep doctor. Andrew was kind of a pit bull by then, ready to chew up any doctor or nurse who gave me any shit. We'd worked through a lot of our own issues since cutting loose from Grace, and he was my ally again.

I was still exhausted most of the time, but slightly less so since I'd started taking CoQ10 supplements. Dr. Saine ordered another sleep study that showed a serious case of what he called periodic restless limb disorder.

"We have several options to treat this," Dr. Saine said. "First, I'd like to check your iron and ferritin levels. If they're low, we can supplement them until they increase. Another option would be to take medication. Gabapentin and clonazepam both have records of success in treating restless legs. I think gabapentin is more effective however."

I hesitated. Not only had my history of adverse drug reactions left me disabled, I'd read reports from people with functional neurological disorder that their symptoms had started during or after exposure to gabapentin.

"I'd rather not take any more drugs, given my history. Let's test my iron and ferritin. If they're low, I'll try supplements first. If supplements don't work, we'll reconvene."

"That sounds like a plan," Dr. Saine agreed.

My ferritin level did turn out to be low, and supplements helped a little. I kicked less as I was trying to go to sleep, but my pedaling legs still woke me throughout the night.

I accepted Dr. Saine's prescription for clonazepam. Within three days of starting it at a dosage of one milligram per night, I sank into a deep depression. By the fifth night, I was in the throes of full-blown suicidal ideation. I hadn't felt suicidal since my hysterectomy.

I told my mind, as I had during the PMDD episodes, that nothing was wrong. But my mind wouldn't listen to reason. I stopped the clonazepam after seven days, and the depression lifted within a week.

I wondered how much of the sadness I'd experienced in the last decade had been because of the benzos that had been cast at me by psychiatrists in an effort to stave off my never-ending anxiety. By the time Dr. Saine prescribed the clonazepam, I'd been almost completely drug free for several months. The only prescription that remained was estradiol. And my mood had been phenomenal. The quickness with which the clonazepam had pushed me into darkness had been astounding.

I scoured my genetic data again and discovered a NAT2 mutation that makes me a slow metabolizer of clonazepam and any other drug processed via the same enzymatic pathway. I shook my head and added this new piece to the puzzle.

I still couldn't hear well. Andrew bought me a captioned phone so I could make appointments for myself again. But I was still functionally deaf in most environments. Sounds oozed together into a giant wall of noise that made speech indecipherable. After several searches, Dr. Google introduced me to the concept of auditory processing disorder.

In February 2016, I arrived for my appointment with renowned audiologist Dr. Jack Katz. In the waiting room, a woman held a screaming baby. With each shriek that left the child's throat, my thoughts became more scattered. I saw motion and aimed my eyes at the short white-haired man walking toward me with his hand extended.

I stood. "Hi, are you Ms. Hiari?" he asked with a smile.

I shook his hand and smiled in return. "Yes," I answered.

"I'm Dr. Katz. Come on back." He gestured down a hallway. Andrew stood and followed us. Dr. Katz turned again and introduced himself to Andrew.

We entered an office. A table extended lengthwise into the middle of the room. Dr. Katz gestured for me to sit across from him and for my husband to sit in a chair against the wall behind me.

"So, what brings you to me?" he asked.

"Um. I've been d-d-diagnosed with hyperacusis, and while I agree with that diagnosis, it doesn't s-s-seem to account for all of the auditory issues I experience. I wanted to find out whether auditory processing disorder could be affecting m-m-me as well."

He nodded. "Okay. I can help you figure that out. What symptoms do you experience?"

"Exposure to sound makes me tired and c-c-confused. The more I hear, the more d-d-difficulty I have finding the words I want to use. I've also noticed that the more exposure I get to sound, the more difficulty I have with my short-term memory. It's like sound somehow makes me forgetful. If I block out sound, I can concentrate and do what I need to d-do, but with exposure, I experience all these c-c-cognitive issues."

He continued to nod. "Have you always had these reactions to sound?"

"Well, I've always been sensitive to sound. For as long as I can remember, I've preferred quiet environments. But I didn't experience this degree of sensitivity until a series of medical treatments I had the year before last." I handed him a folder. "In here are my hearing test results. I've also included a copy of my neuropsychological testing results that document impaired memory and reduced cognitive functioning following exposure to several drugs."

He accepted the papers and began to leaf through them. "Why were you on amitriptyline?"

I took a breath and tried to figure out how to make the long story short. "I had a hormone- based mood d-disorder called premenstrual dysphoric disorder. For years it was misdiagnosed as regular d-depression, so instead of getting the most effective treatment for PMDD, I was just prescribed loads of SSRIs, SNRIs, and eventually amitriptyline. I also had ECT t-t-treatment. I noticed my hearing f-first changed while I was having ECT."

"What's ECT?" he asked.

"It's electroconvulsive therapy. It's where a psy-psy-psychiatrist administers shocks to your b-brain to help with treatment resistant depression."

I watched Dr. Katz's eyes widen. "How do they administer the shocks?"

"They put electrodes on your head. It h-h-happens while you're under anesthesia."

"Do you have any ringing in your ears?"

"I never d-d-did until the ECT. I didn't find out until I s-s-saw Dr. Fluké that it's called *musical tinnitus*. The musical s-sounds transformed into a single high-pitched tone sometime late in 2014. That's all I have now—the high-pitched tone in my left ear."

I watched his brows go up again. "So, this P-M—I'm sorry, what's it called?"

"PMDD."

"This PMDD, do you still experience it?" he asked.

"No, it was cured by a hysterectomy in D-December of 2014."

He asked me a few more questions about my habits and behaviors as a child. I explained how I'd started skipping school in eighth grade.

"What did you do instead of going to school?" No one had ever asked me that before; instead, they'd made assumptions.

"Um, I went to the library and just hung out there. If I couldn't get to the library, I'd hole up somewhere else and read. Basically, I just read, I guess. Sometimes, I'd hang out with a friend, and we'd listen to music and talk." I felt the clarity returning to my speech as time elapsed from the trigger of the baby's cry in the waiting room.

"Thank you for bringing these documents. Let's go ahead and start the testing." He stood up and handed a small binder to Andrew. "This is so you can follow along with the testing, sir. I'm going to play some words and ask you to repeat them. I'm going to play them into each ear separately, and then I'm going to play them into both ears together. Do you have any questions for me before we start?"

I reached up and removed the plugs from my ears. Thankfully, the sounds from the waiting area couldn't be heard back here. The only sound that stood out was the ticking of a clock on the wall. I rested my hands in my lap. "No, no questions."

Over the course of the next several minutes, I listened to and tried to repeat words and phonemes that came through the headphones. After I'd responded to a particularly challenging word, Dr. Katz paused.

"What are you doing when there's a delay before you answer?" he asked. His voice was kind.

I'd experienced similar delays during Dr. Bland's testing, but she hadn't seemed to notice. I'd always had to pause before responding to speech. Dr. Katz was the first person to ask me about it.

"I'm going through all the spelling variations of what I hear to find the most likely candidate," I answered.

"That explains why you're looking up after each sound," he said. "Try to use your visual skills less, and just repeat what you hear."

"You mean, like what I *really* hear, and not what I know the word is *supposed* to be?"

"Yes. Exactly."

"I'll try my best. I've always spelled out everything, so that's going to be quite the adjustment. But I'll try my best."

"Just do what you can. I don't want you to feel too pressured,"

Dr. Katz assured me.

When I stopped spelling the words in my head, I realized that the sounds he was playing weren't English. I repeated what I heard to the best of my ability, but the sounds coming from my mouth were foreign.

"Ooh-uhl," I said.

"What was that word?" he asked.

"I don't know really. *Ooh-uhl* is what it sounded like."

"The word was *wool*," he explained. He placed cards in front of me that offered the spelling.

"Oh. I never would've guessed that unless we were talking about sheep or sweaters."

"Good. That's good! You're using your visual skills less. That gives me more information."

After a few more minutes of this, he asked me how I was feeling. "I'm exhausted."

"When you don't hear things correctly, your brain has to do a lot of extra work. That will make you tired. We can stop for today and finish in our next session. May I ask what's the reason for your unusual mouth movement?"

"Um, yeah. One neurologist I saw, Dr. Wise, he called it an oral dyskinesia. It onset after I was overdosed on amitriptyline."

He made a note, then stood to see us out. "It was very nice meeting both of you. I'll see you next week."

I said goodbye and inserted my earplugs as Andrew and I headed toward the lobby.

"Thank God he wasn't an ass," cheered Andrew once we were in the car.

"Yes," I agreed.

---

I continued to see Dr. Katz and learned more about my brain's responses to speech.

"You paused again before answering. Why did you do that?" he asked again after another set of exercises.

"Well, I went to answer, but I could tell that the words that were going to come out of my mouth were nonsense words, not the words I was thinking of. Sometimes there's a disconnect—it's hard to explain—so I took a breath and rearranged the letters in my head, so that my speech would be clearer. If I can't think to rearrange the letters and words, I just talk nonsense—or I can't talk at all."

It felt strange explaining these inner workings of my mind. I'd always assumed they were normal.

He nodded. "Well, that wraps up our testing," he said a few minutes later. "Can I ask you a few more questions?"

"Sure."

"Did you have a lot of middle ear infections, particularly in your first year of life?"

"Um, I'm not sure about ear infections, but I've been told I had pneumonia and other respiratory issues before I was one."

"Okay. When they did this ECT, where did they place the electrodes?"

I pointed to my forehead. "They did it two ways. Sometimes they put electrodes above each of my eyebrows. They called that bifrontal. Most of the time, though, they put one above my right eyebrow and one further back on my head." I pointed to a spot between my forehead and the crown of my head.

The expression on Dr. Katz's face was nothing short of horrified. I watched him try to suppress it when he saw that I had returned my gaze from my hands to his face.

"Please take care of yourself, Ms. Hiari. I'll have my report ready for you when I see you next week."

Several days later, I returned.

"You clearly have auditory processing disorder. I think it's probably more severe than my initial testing shows due to your age and the extent of your use of coping mechanisms. But even for what we could confirm with my tests, yours is quite severe. There are four types of APD: Decoding, which is the ability to quickly and accurately digest speech; Tolerance-Fading Memory, which is the combination of poor understanding of speech in noise as well as difficulty with short-term auditory memory; Organization, which is the ability to organize one's thoughts and maintain proper sequence; and Integration, which is difficulty bringing information together. You have three of the four types of APD. You definitely have issues with Decoding, Tolerance-Fading Memory, and Integration. I cannot rule out Organization as a possible component at this time, nor can I confirm it. We'll find out whether that plays a role after we start your therapy."

I struggled to take down notes as he spoke. I couldn't make sense of all of it, and I had a lifelong habit of pretending to understand when I didn't. I caught myself. I could ask for repetition here. Dr. Katz would understand. So, I asked for repetition until I understood, and as I'd predicted, Dr. Katz remained patient.

"From what you've told me, it's clear you've had APD for most, if not all, of your life. You've developed visual coping mechanisms to offset the disadvantages the APD presents. I think the ECT exacerbated the severity of your auditory processing issues and compromised your coping mechanisms. The placement of the electrodes corresponds exactly to the parts of the brain where certain categories of APD are understood to be situated. We audiologists have thought for some time that the center for speech in noise difficulty is the anterior lobe, and that corresponds with the ECT electrode placement. That, and your experience of musical tinnitus during the treatment, make me certain that's what happened."

I dropped my face into my hands as my tears poured. Hard coughs caught in my throat. Memories flashed through my head like cars on a passing train: Sitting in hallways or skipping school because of how I'd become confused and overwhelmed by sounds in classrooms. Refusing to cross cafeteria thresholds because I couldn't withstand the onslaught of all of the voices. Requesting a hearing test in college because I couldn't understand my professors.

I'd once spent days fretting over whether I should ask an English professor for an alternate assignment. The professor had instructed us to write about a film. I'd figured out by then that movies made no sense to me. In the end, I'd ended up not talking to the professor about it. I didn't think he'd believe me. I'd never heard of anyone else having a problem understanding movies. I worried that he'd think I was lazy and trying to get out of an assignment. I'd written about the film and accepted my grade of D. If I'd been allowed to write about a book, my grade would've likely been an A.

At my job at the grocery store, I could never hear over the meat slicers, chicken fryers, or bread-slicing machines. I was constantly asking customers to repeat their orders, and I was forever being yelled at when I asked for repetition.

Years later, when I'd worked office jobs, I'd often asked to have my desk moved because I couldn't think if I was seated next to a coworker with a loud voice.

I thought of my hatred of radio shows that played sounds during news stories. I thought of my lifelong inability to speak in groups because I couldn't keep up when multiple people were talking. I thought of my inability to interject because the moment of opportunity passed by too quickly.

There'd been the cascade of insults that had fallen around me for as long as I could remember: "Are you just gonna stand there and look pretty?" "For somebody who's supposed to be smart, you sure act stupid." "It's so funny how you pronounce that word!" "You talk like you're stoned!"

Hot tears leaked from between my fingers that were still pressed against my face.

"Ms. Hiari? Are you all right?" came Dr. Katz's voice.

"I'm sorry. It's just—it's just." I wiped my tears with my sleeve. "I'm sorry."

"I understand." He looked sad. "The only worse thing that I could imagine is seeing this happen to your child—"

"Okay, doctor. I'm sorry about that," I said. He looked more upset than I felt. I didn't want him to feel sad. "Please continue. I'll be alright."

"If you're sure . . . I don't want to push you—"

"No, no. I just had to move through some feelings. Don't worry. I don't have a mood disorder anymore. I just get sad and then move on like a regular person now," I tried to assure him.

It took him a moment to continue. He seemed to be trying to sort out whether what he had to say would hurt me again.

"Most people have what we call binaural symmetry—" he started.

"Would you spell that please?" I interrupted. He did, and I scribbled it in my notebook.

"What that means is the sounds you hear with your left ear and the sounds you hear with your right ear are supposed to be identical when they meet in the middle in your brain. The right ear has a more direct path to the auditory center. The left ear's path isn't quite as direct, and on its way to the center, it has time to pick up more noise or interference, so to speak. Your left ear is picking up far more noise than is typical. By the time your signals meet in the middle, instead of matching, they're different. You don't have binaural symmetry. You have to do extra work to reconcile the signals. That's called Integration. It's the most challenging presentation of APD."

Andrew hadn't been able to come to my follow-up visit with Dr. Katz. When he came home from work, I explained the details of my diagnosis to him. "This is why I can't stand being interrupted by phone calls throughout the day. It disrupts my concentration far more than it would the concentration of a regular person."

After nine years of begging for peace, Andrew finally stopped calling me throughout the day.

*With your auditory processing disorder diagnosis, things were really starting to make sense. Did you think you had solved the mystery of what had happened to your brain?*

Huh? Yeah, I thought that for like a minute. Then something else happened. But before we get to that, do you realize what else had happened in this time frame? No? I'll tell you then. I got my diagnosis from Dr. Katz on February 26, 2016. My ECT had started on April 23, 2014. The first record I can find that documents my musical tinnitus is on April 30, 2014. I got Andrew to call a few lawyers for me. Do you remember how nobody wanted to take my case back when all I had was the tardive dyskinesia diagnosis? This time the lawyers all said they'd want my case if it wasn't for the statute issue.

I was screwed. Nobody wanted my case because nobody had time to prepare. Every penny I'd have to pay to repair my brain and auditory system would be paid for by me and Andrew, which really meant paid by Andrew, insurance companies, and an SSDI system that shouldn't have to pay for the outcome of physician and pharmaceutical-induced injuries.

# CHAPTER THIRTY-ONE

THE COOL MARCH air flowed over my cheeks. I gripped the handlebars and pedaled. I saw the mud and leaned left. The front tire hit the mud, and the bike slid out from under me. Bam! I went down hard on my side, crushing my arm beneath me.

It was a three-mile walk back to the car. Even worse than the long walk and the pain in my left wrist was the crunching sound that emanated from the injury with each step. I could hear the crunching in the same way I still heard my blood pumping in my ears.

"Let's go to Local Hospital. It's closest," Andrew suggested.

"No. Local Hospital's records say I have borderline personality disorder and conversion disorder. I'll get treated like shit. Let's go to Prairie Wind Regional. I've made it this long; a few extra minutes won't kill me."

I'd sent a request to Dr. Thueban and Local Hospital asking that the borderline personality disorder diagnosis be removed from my records and replaced with a diagnosis of premenstrual dysphoric disorder (resolved). I'd included a letter from Grace that concurred with my assertion that I'd never met the criteria for a borderline diagnosis.

I hadn't been surprised when my request had been denied. And I knew it meant I'd never receive unprejudiced treatment at Local Hospital.

After we arrived at Prairie Wind Regional, I was quickly taken back to a treatment room. Andrew explained my auditory needs to each staff person who entered the room. "My wife's very sensitive to sound. Please keep your voices low, and speak one at a time. If you start talking too loudly, or if you all start talking at once, she'll become confused."

The doctor spoke slowly and enunciated so that I could understand him. He faced me so that I could see his mouth. There was no confusion. There were no tears. He put me in a splint and sent me on my way after X-rays revealed I'd fractured my distal radius.

I followed up with an orthopedic surgeon. "You're lucky to have such a clean break," Dr. Ossein said. "I expect it'll heal quickly. You definitely won't need surgery."

Two weeks later, I was back. My forearm had swollen so immensely that the cast could barely enclose it. My wedding ring choked my plump finger. I wore earplugs under gigantic 3M Peltor X-series muffs as a tech sawed away the cast and replaced it with a fresh one. I returned a few days later because the swelling had persisted and the cast had begun to cut off my circulation again.

"You must be part of a very small group of people whose bodies can't tolerate casting," the physician assistant told me. "We'll put you back in a splint. That'll work fine."

I endured the agony of the whining saw for another cast removal. I returned a few weeks later. After another X-ray, Dr. Ossein told me the bone had healed. "You can resume your normal activities," he said. I smiled. Normal activities meant typing with both hands.

I was surprised by the changes to my forearm, wrist, and hand. Hair had grown in patches where none had ever grown before. It even grew in places on my hand the cast hadn't been in contact with.

The area near the ulna was still swollen, even though the fracture had been on the opposite side. Deep-blue bruising came and went at the former fracture site for no reason I could discern.

*That sounds painful, but what does it have to do with your other issues?*

Well, I started looking for a way to treat the inflammation from the fracture. Ibuprofen gives me hives, so I looked for an alternative. Turmeric with black pepper kept coming up in my searches, so Andrew went out and bought some. Guess what? It didn't do anything for my wrist, but my hyperacusis got way better! Things seemed less loud within a few days of my first dose.

And you know what else happened? The weird mouth movement disappeared. And my nighttime confusion and paranoia became less frequent. I usually got confused—I don't know, four or five nights a week? Regardless of sound, I got this onset of confusion after dinner. With the turmeric, that got cut back to one or two nights a week.

Within a week of starting the turmeric complex, I went from wearing foam earplugs all the time to wearing light earplugs. I could walk in the park again. I still couldn't walk past the screaming kids on the playground unless I switched back to the foam plugs—but it was a huge improvement. I still had to wear my Bose to places that played music or had lots of people talking, but I could leave the house way more often than before. So, I got really hopeful, and I started making plans to get out more and do more things.

Because of my response to the enhanced bioavailability turmeric, I wondered if my hyperacusis and cognitive problems had been a byproduct of inflammation in my brain and auditory system. And if they were, I wondered what was causing the inflammation.

But that reminds me of something else that happened before the turmeric miracle. I'd been taking calcium and magnesium supplements on the advice of Dr. Fahrig. One week in mid-2015, I'd forgotten to put them in my supplement tray. After just one week without them, my cognition had improved tremendously. I experimented with it. I went back and forth with and without the calcium and magnesium. Turns out there was definitely a causal relationship. Something about calcium and magnesium at that dosage, or by that delivery system, wasn't meshing with my brain.

**You said you started to make plans to get out and do more. What were your plans?**

Well, the first thing I did was apply for a residency program at a Buddhist retreat center. I thought I'd learn some new meditation techniques and see if I could harness the power of my brain to heal itself. I let the facilities manager know up front about my auditory issues, and I asked if they could accommodate me. The manager said they'd try to make it work.

I got ready for my trip out East. And I thought that while I was out there, I should visit an immunologist to get their take on whether I had any immune or autoimmune issues. I scheduled to see an immunologist at the University of Virginia who was familiar with mast cell disease. That's where Dr. Google had been leading me—toward a mast cell disorder.

Before my appointment, I asked my primary care PA to order some labs—tryptase, prostaglandins, and leukotrienes. All those are kinda esoteric tests associated with mast cell disease.

**What did the tests show?**

Hold on, hold on, I'll get to that. I only lasted two weeks out East. The acoustics at the retreat center were rough. The room where the staff meetings were held was awful. The floor was wood, the walls were paneled, and every single sound echoed. Voices overlapped, and I'd get confused. The folks out there, they tried to make it work. They put down rugs on the floor to help absorb the sound. They spoke one at a time. But I just couldn't freaking hear!

When I arrived there, only a handful of staff members were present and it was pretty quiet. I could walk around without any hearing protection a lot of the time because we were up on a mountain, away from city sounds. Unless somebody was mowing the grass or weed eating or whatever—then I'd wear earmuffs. But as more people came for the big summer retreat, it got louder and more chaotic.

So, you know, with all that going on, I had to be realistic. I told my supervisors I had to leave. My ears and brain just weren't ready.

Andrew had driven out with me so that I could have my car out there. I thought that before I went home, I'd stop in DC to visit Gallaudet and check out a couple of museums.

**Who's Gallaudet?**

Huh? Gallaudet University is the only university in the country designed for deaf and hard of hearing students. It's a bilingual school. They teach in American Sign Language—ASL—and English. As soon as I'd learned I had auditory processing disorder, I'd headed to the real experts. You remember how I told you that the only people who stood by me after I started criticizing health care culture were people with disabilities? Well, I knew if anybody had advice on how to navigate life with different hearing, or no hearing at all, it would be Deaf and hard of hearing people. I'd signed up for sign language lessons with a deaf tutor, and as soon as I started learning, I realized ASL felt natural. I also realized that when my brain got confused and I couldn't speak, I could still sign. The neural pathways to my hands still worked.

DC was loud. That part didn't surprise me—it's a big city. But they have a honking fetish out there. They use their horns for everything. The sun came up—honkkkk! You cut me off—honkkkk! I forgot to put on deodorant—honkkkk! I mean, it's ridiculous! But with my Bose and my plugs, I managed to get through the honking and find parking. From there I took the train into the city. I got to Gallaudet—miraculously—because there are very few visual cues on the subway. I had to count the stops to find the right place. Thank goodness I could count that day!

It was a sunny day, warm and comfortable with a breeze. The trees were lush and green. My brain was focused. Everything was perfect. I put my earplugs in as I prepared to walk off the quiet campus and back into honking land. Then my phone rang, which was odd. The few people in my life knew I only used my captioned home phone for calls now.

The caller ID said *Burt*, which was even stranger. I plugged in my Bose and answered the call.

"May I speak to Twilah please?" a woman asked.

"Yes, speaking."

"Hi, this is blah-blah. Blah-blah—I'm sorry to tell you your dad passed away in his sleep last night."

"Oh, I'm so sorry to hear that," I said to the woman. I hadn't caught her name. I realized I was offering sympathy to her when she expected I'd be the one to be upset. But if she'd known right away that Burt had died, she'd been closer to him than I'd been.

"It's okay. I'm just calling his kids—"

I couldn't follow. Traffic buzzed around me. "Um, I'm actually in Washington, DC, right now. It'll take me awhile to get back, at least a couple of days. But I'll leave right away. When's the service?"

"We don't know yet."

"Okay. I'll head back now."

※

I checked my email in the morning. My lab results were there. The tryptase and leukotrienes were normal. But the prostaglandin E2 was high at 1006. A normal range is 400-620. I had no idea what that meant.

I'd canceled my appointment at UVA when I left the retreat center. I put the question about the lab results behind me as I drove into the green hills of Maryland. Other than eating salads from convenience stores, I fasted the entire drive home. I'd figured out that most foods exacerbated my confusion and caused abdominal pain, diarrhea, and hot flashes. I wanted to stay lucid, as well as pain and diarrhea free. My food strategy worked, and my mind stayed clear enough to drive. A few days later, I was back in Kansas.

※

Jeffrey fought back tears as the urn was lowered into the ground. As far as we knew, Burt had been his biological father. Their relationship had been rocky.

Burt had married my mother in 1961. In 1966, she gave birth to Glen. My mother had confessed to me in 2014 that Burt wasn't Glen's father. I wondered if Burt had ever known that. Glen hadn't known until I'd written him with the news. At age fifty, Glen had learned that Burt wasn't his dad. My mother had excused her lie about my paternity by saying she'd never figured out the right time to tell me. In fifty years, my mother had evidently never found the right time to tell Glen.

Between 1966 and 1988, Burt had provided materially for Glen and then me, when I was born in 1975—the two bastard children of his wife's affairs. I was grateful he'd done so, but there was no feeling attached to this gratitude, just an abstract idea of thankfulness.

I watched as the children and family of Burt's partner, Patricia, who'd died the year before, arrived in shorts and dirty boots, low-cut shirts, and skintight jeans. They talked loudly and joked about things that had nothing to do with Burt as soon as the urn was placed in the ground. Burt seemed to have meant little to the people he'd surrounded himself with in the years following his divorce from my mom.

*Had he ever been the center of anyone's world?*

The question brought dampness to my eyes, but it stopped short of forming a tear.

I reached into my mind and tried to uncover fond memories of my stepfather. There were none. It was at that point that a tear formed in the corner of my eye. How very sad for a person to leave this earth and have no one who truly mourns him.

# CHAPTER THIRTY-TWO

I RETURNED TO my obsession. The physician assistant was supposed to have ordered a test for prostaglandin D2, which is a mast cell product. But she'd accidentally ordered prostaglandin E2, which is not a mast cell product. I looked up PGE2 and learned that it's associated with inflammation. Some articles tied it specifically to neuroinflammation. It came up in relationship to autism and Alzheimer's in several articles. But the stuff I found was hard to read. It was technical neurology stuff, way beyond the scope of what I could understand given the impaired state of my brain.

I looked at all my unusual health metrics. My alkaline phosphatase, a liver enzyme, had been high between 2014 and 2015, but had returned to a normal range by 2016, when I'd stopped all my medications.

Six months after the fracture, I still had bruising in my wrist that came and went without any triggers I could identify. I thought of the long list of dermatological, gastrointestinal, and neurological reactions I'd had to foods, smells, and other things in the environment. My genetic tests showed I had JAK2 mutations associated with myeloproliferative disorders.

A Google search for myeloproliferative disorders took me to Canada's Mastocytosis Society website. I was back to the mast cells my original search had led me to. As I read, I realized that mastocytosis was even broader in scope than functional neurological disorder. That would've made me skeptical, but the key difference between mastocytosis and FND was that mastocytosis posited a cause first and explained how symptoms followed from the cause, while the researchers of FND had nothing better than guesses in regard to causation.

According to the Mastocytosis Society, I presently or previously had a lot of symptoms that corresponded with the disease: skin rash, hives, fatigue, flushing and severe sweating, bone pain, chemical reactions, difficult menses, persistent diarrhea, cognitive impairment, swelling and inflammation, odd reactions to insect stings, temperature sensitivity, anaphylactoid reactions, gastrointestinal pain, bloating, unexplained medication reactions, frequent urination, recurring infections, constipation, unexplained bruising, and tinnitus or hearing problems.

If I was experiencing mast-cell-induced inflammation, I didn't want to keep throwing supplements at it if I could learn dietary or lifestyle modifications that would address the root cause of my problems. Turmeric had started to lose its effectiveness anyway. I now had to take two or three times as much to get the results I'd gotten originally. My sensitivity to sound was increasing in severity and so was the screaming tinnitus in my left ear. And I was losing my speech again.

~⚘~

In July 2016, I saw a local immunologist, Dr. Mermer. The appointment didn't start off well. My captioned phone was hard to use—there was a long lag before I'd see the words, so I'd made the appointment using the relay system for deaf and hard of hearing people. I'd asked via relay if Dr. Mermer diagnosed and treated mast cell disease, and the receptionist had assured me he did. But when I arrived, the receptionist said I'd been scheduled for an asthma evaluation. Using my notes, and struggling with my speech again, I did my best to explain to him how I'd had gamma globulin injections as a baby and how I'd suffered anaphylaxis after being stung by an insect in a park. Dr. Mermer wrote in my chart that I had hypogammaglobulinemia and an allergy to insect venom. He ordered bloodwork, then raged at me when he read the results.

"Blah-grrr-blah. There's nothing wrong with your gamma globulin level. Why did you tell me you had a gamma globulin problem? And you have no insect allergy! Grrr-blah-blah." He stood up and started pacing. His face was now bright red. When he sat back down, I could understand him better.

"I'll give you a pneumonia vaccine," he said. "You need a pneumonia vaccine. You need to take Pepcid. You're just having acid reflux. There's nothing else wrong. You have no immune deficiency. But your B12 is high, much too high, and your B6 too! Your B6 is three times normal! Are you getting B12 injections? I saw your supplement list! *Patients like you with your supplements and your injections!*"

"Huh? I've never had a buh-B12 injection, and I don't take a B12 supplement. And, and, I'm uh, uh vegetarian, s-s-o I don't get it from meat."

"Sure, sure. Whatever, whatever. Take this Pepcid, and see me in two weeks."

Two weeks later, I was back. "I stopped taking the Pepcid because it gave me really bad pain in my Achilles tendons. I had the same pain with lamotrigine and a cholesterol drug—"

Dr. Mermer started mumbling and shaking his head again. "If you stop these medicines after an extremely short time, we'll never know anything! You don't just stop medicines when your doctor tells you to take them!"

"But it hurt my tendons *really* bad. I could b-barely walk."

He huffed and puffed and muttered some more. I left his office and never went back.

I got very sick after the pneumonia vaccine. I started to feel dizzy when I'd transition from lying to sitting to standing. I developed something called orthostatic hypotension, which is a sign of injury to the autonomic nervous system.

I told Dr. Saine that my brain problems were getting worse again and how they were triggered by allergic reactions. This was a huge problem because I was now having reactions to everything—the scents of cleaning products in public bathrooms, the dust swirling up from the dry summer streets, the scents some people wore at the Buddhist temple, the only place I still went besides doctors' offices.

Dr. Saine ordered a lumbar puncture. After the radiologist drew my spinal fluid, I felt great. My speech and thoughts became clearer. My hyperacusis got better too, kind of like when I first started taking turmeric. And I could understand speech more easily.

*That's incredible. How did a lumbar puncture do that?*

I might've had something called intracranial hypertension or IH, which is elevated cerebrospinal fluid pressure. But since that wasn't on Dr. Saine's radar, he hadn't ordered a pressure measurement. IH would mean that my spinal fluid was compressing my brain. Some research shows that IH occurs more often in women with a history of menstrual dysfunction. Interesting, huh? IH can cause visual problems too. But intracranial hypertension isn't the only reason a lumbar puncture could've helped me.

*What would've caused intracranial hypertension?*

IH can be caused by brain injuries, adverse drug reactions, hormonal issues, and obesity. It seems some people are genetically predisposed to it. Elevated cerebrospinal fluid pressure totally corresponds with how Mom said her head "blew up." Lots of women say their IH fluctuates with barometric pressure.

*That's a huge breakthrough. That must feel very validating.*

Yeah, it was. So, I scheduled to see another immunologist. This one, Dr. Rekon, was at a research hospital. He ordered even more blood tests than Dr. Mermer had. His tests showed that my B and T cells were very elevated, which made Andrew think my body was responding to an infection. But Dr. Rekon said the results were nothing to worry about because it meant I didn't have an immune deficiency. You surprised by that? Well, wait, the story isn't over yet.

Dr. Rekon actually communicated. He didn't dismiss my complaints. He taught me about this concept of the microbiome. The microbiome consists of the microorganisms that live on us and in us; it also means the genomes of those microorganisms. If your microbiome isn't healthy, you aren't healthy.

"When people have diverse microbiomes, like you still see in traditional indigenous populations, those people don't get the diseases we get here in the West. There's no cancer, no heart disease, and no autoimmune disorders. In modern industrialized countries, we have very little microbial diversity, and that allows us to be affected by a lot of problems you don't see in traditional aboriginal populations," Dr. Rekon said.

After my appointment, I'd gone online and started reading more about the microbiome. The more I read, the more things made sense. Some researchers have uncovered evidence that suggests autism is associated with the microbes in our gut.

We get some of our microbiome in utero. Babies aren't completely sterile like people used to think. After we've stewed in the uterus and picked up some organisms there, we get more organisms when we're born. The quality of our mother's microbiome before and during pregnancy, and her toxic load, matter a lot. The microbes we get also depend on if we're delivered vaginally or by C-section. The development continues based on factors such as whether we're breast or bottle fed. Thirty percent of the beneficial bacteria in a baby's intestinal tract comes from breast milk, and 10 percent or more comes from the skin on the mother's breast.

Every environmental interaction from that point forward sculpts and changes our microbiome. Because of how these organisms are transferred from person to person, via food, grooming—all kinds of things—our environment ends up being almost as big an influence on our health as our genetics. Stress can affect our microbiome too. It can make physical changes to it. That's how stress can cause physical illness.

I had far fewer episodes of illness when my diet and exercise routines were in good shape, but then you all started to fuck up my delicate balance by adding in all those psych drugs. I didn't have the ability to metabolize them or the microbial fortitude to withstand them. The drugs made me gain weight, and my fat new body had distorted cravings. When my diet mutated to sugar laden and calorically excessive, I lost even more of my protective microbiota. Going into 2014, my gut was already fucked up. I was primed for a massive malfunction.

Do you know what can screw up our microbiome really bad? Antibiotics. They can wipe out damn near everything good in your gut. Then you're left with no defenses. Your immune system can't do its job without the power of a healthy microbiome behind it.

Prolonged use of bacterial antibiotics like vancomycin causes mitochondrial dysfunction and oxidative damage to our cells. Mitochondria are the energy centers of our cells. They're the primary place where oxygen consumption occurs in our bodies. They house an enormous range of antioxidants and detoxifying enzymes. An important one of these is glutathione. Glutathione is a peptide or protein. Most enzymes are peptides. Glutathione is also a neuropeptide and a neurotransmitter, which means neurons use it to communicate with each other. Glutathione bonds with drugs and helps us metabolize them. It's the body's master detoxification enzyme. It helps protect us against oxidative damage, and it plays a role in the production of leukotrienes. The massive amounts of vancomycin I'd taken for the C. diff had exacerbated the mitochondrial and glutathione dysfunction I'd probably had my entire life. That had made it even harder for me to metabolize the medications that were still being thrown at me. It also disrupted my energy production, which led to more problems with wakefulness and sleep. That's why I started to have more energy after I added CoQ10 to my supplement list. CoQ10 supports mitochondrial function. It's also an antioxidant.

Long-term use of bacterial antibiotics also causes damage to cellular membrane lipids. A lipid is a fatty acid. Prostaglandin E2—you remember how that marker was elevated? PGE2 is a lipid that's produced from a substance called arachidonic acid in cellular membranes. PGE2 and leukotrienes are lipid mediators, and they're also markers of oxidative stress. There's research that shows altered function of fatty acid metabolic pathways of autistics. Other studies show elevated PGE2 and leukotrienes in autistics, which would be one possible outcome of misbehaving metabolic pathways.

Our gut is our second brain. Do you know that? It has its own neural network called the enteric nervous system. The chemicals and networks found in our guts are parallel to those found in our brains. I had my gut microbes mapped and sure enough, I had virtually no microbial diversity.

Dr. Rekon told me to eat local food that was non-GMO and hadn't been chemically treated and to take probiotics to add some diversity back into my gut. He said he couldn't recommend anything more specific because the specifics of what I'd been experiencing didn't correspond to any diagnosis he was aware of.

After I got home, I downloaded a book he'd recommended on nutrition, and I realized my diet didn't look anything like the diet in the book. I'd been a vegetarian for religious reasons and also because I'd read lots of books that purported a plant-based diet as the healthiest way to eat. But the book Dr. Rekon recommended was backed by far more research than the books I'd read before, and it recommended a diet filled with high-quality animal proteins and vegetables that could be eaten uncooked. It said that beans and grains cause inflammation, and grains and beans had been the backbone of my diet. I also learned that grains and beans are high in histamines, and histamines are one of the most powerful engines behind allergies and allergylike responses in the body.

It was a big mental shift, but Andrew went out and bought some local grass-fed beef. So, I added meat to my diet, and I stopped eating beans and grains. I added in more leafy greens and raw and roasted vegetables. With these changes, I immediately had less flushing, fewer hot flashes, and less diarrhea. The head pressure that had gone away after the lumbar puncture stayed gone, and my meltdowns became less frequent.

I used to have these brief spikes of anger about an hour after eating breakfast every day, and every time I'd have them, I'd sit down to meditate until the anger went away. Well, when I transitioned from a breakfast of steel-cut oatmeal to a pea protein shake with coconut-almond milk and a handful of blueberries, those daily spikes of anger disappeared. A little more experimentation and observation confirmed that my anger only came on after eating meals high in carbohydrates or histamines. Pretty cool, huh?

༄

The next immunologist I saw dug in a different direction.

"I had gamma globulin injections between the ages of three and five," I explained. "My family says I had some kind of immune deficiency, but I don't remember having a lot of reactions or infections until I got older, like in my late teens. The tests Dr. Mermer and Dr. Rekon did don't show any deficiencies, so I don't understand why I needed the injections."

"Some children are born with a gamma globulin deficiency that resolves on its own by age five. I'm not at all surprised you're no longer deficient," Dr. Foster said. "I think you could have mast cell activation disorder. It's never my first choice for a diagnosis, but if you've ruled everything else out and you still have symptoms like yours, mast cell activation is the term we use to explain them. We'll start treatment with ten milligrams of Zyrtec daily, then follow up with me in eight weeks."

Andrew brought home a bottle of generic Zyrtec. Within an hour of taking the first pill, my chest had become tight, my breathing had become shallow, and my lips had started to itch. I'd gone to the ER, where they gave me a breathing treatment, steroids, and IV Benadryl. I'd reacted to an antihistamine!

I didn't go back to that doctor because she refused to believe I had a reaction to Zyrtec. Dr. Foster asked me to come into her office and do a challenge where she'd give me small doses of Zyrtec over time and watch how I reacted. Well, since so many of my allergic reactions have serious effects on my brain, I didn't want to take her challenge. It sounded dangerous. I did some more reading, chatted with some other mast cell activation patients online, and saw yet another immunologist.

Dr. Cumen shook his head as he flipped through my medical records. "Functional neurological disorder?" he asked with a small laugh. "Is that what neurologists call it when they can't figure out that an injury to your immune system is affecting your brain?"

"Ha-ha! You get it!" I said.

"Yeah," he replied, still rifling through the pages. "You get urinary urgency and frequency with your allergic reactions? That's detrusor dysfunction, which goes along with the other brain and central nervous system involvement. Ah, and fixed-drug eruptions to your skin? Yes—all of your symptoms make sense in the context of mast cell activation, but it isn't a diagnosis most doctors are familiar with yet. And at the bigger institutions, they only treat patients with systemic mastocytosis that can be quantified through high tryptase levels—that's the only mast cell mediator they'll measure. But that's very limiting, because there are hundreds of different mediators released by mast cells. Your tryptase levels are normal. Tryptase levels can be normal even with very severe mast cell disease. I think I can help you. Have you ever tried oral cromolyn for your symptoms?"

"No." I shook my head.

"Benzodiazepines are mast cell stabilizers too—" he started.

"Oh no. I can't tolerate benzos. They make me suicidal," I interjected.

"I wonder if that's the actual benzo or if one of the excipients in the drug makes you feel that way? Well, we have lots of options for treating this, but it'll be a trial and error process. I can't promise quick results. We'll have to experiment with different treatments, but I think we can get somewhere. It may be a year or more before we find the right drug combination that works for you."

*Benzodiazepines are mast cell stabilizers? Do you think it's possible that despite the side effects, they kept you from having more serious reactions while you were on them?*

You're finally figuring out how to think through these things, aren't you, Doc? Yes, I absolutely think that. The same drugs that made me hallucinate and want to die probably kept me from having a whole lot of other reactions.

In July 2017, we drove to Minnesota to see mast cell activation disorder pioneer Dr. Lawrence Afrin. Dr. Afrin read the nine-page history I'd composed and skimmed through the 600 pages of medical records that accompanied it.

He added a few new questions to the exam repertoire that I was now well accustomed to. "Have you had any problems with your eyes or vision? Do you have times when it seems like your eyes can't focus?" he asked.

"Yes."

"How about your hair? Anything you've noticed there?"

"Yes, like now." I reached up and touched a small chunk of wooly curls. "I have this crop of short new patches, so it must have gone through a falling-out phase earlier this year that I didn't notice. That happens a lot, and I usually can't figure out what causes it."

"How about your nails?"

I extended my right hand. "This thumbnail split years ago, and I have no idea why. It's been split since. I never injured it or anything."

"Mmm-hmm. Cracked and ridged too, I see," he said before typing more notes. Then he said, "Let's take a look at your mouth. Do you get sores in your mouth?"

"Yes. All the time. They come and go."

I opened wide and stuck out my tongue. He shined a light into the cavity.

"Looks like your dentist has had a lot of fun with you," he said.

"Yeah, I have cavities every time I go. Dentists have always told me it makes no sense considering I have really good oral hygiene. I've had two root canals too."

He examined my skin, scratching his nails over it as Dr. Cumen had done. "You really light up, don't you?" he asked as he looked at the patch of skin he'd scratched, which was now bright red and inflamed. After I'd moved back to a chair from the exam table, he spoke again.

"Your history is textbook mast cell disease. I always ask who first suspected this could be mast cell related. You? Your husband? One of your doctors?"

"Me."

He nodded. "That's usually the case."

"I have a question," I interjected. "Do you think premenstrual dysphoric disorder is a presentation of mast cell disease?"

"Well, I can't prove it, but I've seen a lot of PMDD and PMS with mast cell disease. It certainly seems like a strong possibility that one cause underlies all of these problems, rather than so many of my patients having been so uniquely unlucky as to have such a long list of unrelated issues."

I nodded. I'd thought the same thing many times. I'd thought the NIH study that had uncovered a rogue gene complex associated with PMDD was only the tip of the iceberg.

"It's nice to have someone look at this differently. I'm tired of being told this is psychogenic," I said after I sorted through those thoughts.

"Somatoform illness?" He chuckled as he made more notes. "That's the one thing you haven't had."

Several weeks later, I read Dr. Afrin's final report. In addition to known mast cell mediators, he'd tested me for polymorphisms related to drug metabolism. I hadn't told Dr. Afrin that I already knew I was a poor metabolizer of several drugs. I needed that documentation added to my medical record from the authoritative perspective of a physician.

I didn't think it was possible to feel validated when reading a medical record, but that's exactly how I felt when I read what

Dr. Afrin had written.

> Kudos to the patient, because I think she's likely right in her suspicion that a mast cell activation disorder (MCAD)—and far more likely the far more prevalent (if only recently recognized) type termed mast cell activation syndrome (MCAS) than the rare (but long recognized) type termed mastocytosis—is at the root of most or all of her chronic multisystem polymorbidity of general themes of inflammation, allergy, and aberrant tissue growth/development. Beyond all the other diseases already ruled out by the great extent of testing she's undergone to date, I don't know of any other human disease that comes anywhere near as close as MCAS does to accounting, directly or indirectly, for the full range and chronicity of all the symptoms and findings here. Of note too, I'm not saying that any of her prior diagnoses are wrong—other than any assertions of psychosomatism which might have been made along the way. It's just that each of them accounts for only one subset or another of all that's gone on in her, while MCAS can account for most or all of everything that's been going on in her.
>
> Addendum (9/4/17): Sometimes persistence pays off: GI tract biopsy reexaminations have resulted and complete the diagnostic picture.
>
> Of note, again, I don't think any of her prior diagnoses are wrong (other than any assertions of psychosomatism that might have been made along the way), but the diagnosis that seems to best underlie/unify the largest portion (potentially even all) of her large array of past and present issues is MCAS, and therefore treatment efforts directed at such would seem to be warranted. To be sure, all of her physicians must maintain vigilance for other processes for which—again, whether ultimately dependent on, or completely

independent of, her MCAS—standard therapies other than mast-cell-directed therapy have been defined, as such standard therapies would of course be the more appropriate choices for such processes. However, with MCAS now having been defined in this patient per published diagnostic criteria, emergence of a new process that is potentially consistent with MCAS can be reasonably attributed to MCAS once other "routine" evaluation for that process has ruled out other "traditional" causes for such a process.

This patient has been found to have poor-metabolizing polymorphisms in CYP2D6 and CYP2C19 (but normal CYP2C9 and CYP3A4), so her physicians and pharmacists should check for potential problems from these polymorphisms with any medication recommended for her in the future, as dosing adjustments—or even complete avoidance of certain drugs—may be needed.

Note medication excipients (e.g., fillers, binders, dyes, preservatives) often are triggers, and rapid adverse reaction to an ordinarily well-tolerated drug in an MCAS patient is less likely a sign of intolerance of the active ingredient and far more likely a sign of an excipient reaction mandating prompt return to the pharmacist (commercial or compounding) to identify alternative formulations to be tried which do not contain any of the offending formulation's excipients. Adding a drug to the allergy list is unhelpful—indeed, frankly counterproductive—when the true offending agent is an excipient in the particular formulations of the drug that were tried. Offending excipients should be identified as specifically as possible, added to the allergy list, screened against the rest of the patient's present medication list, and screened against all medications prescribed in the future.

Addendum (9/15/2017): I received results of additional CD117 restaining of prior biopsies . . . from 12/24/14 . . .

the myometrium [smooth tissue of the uterus] definitely showed increased mast cells at 30-40/hpf.

─✣─

This takes us back to the microbiome. Do you know that a huge part of your immune system is in your GI tract? The destruction of my microbiome exacerbated the malfunction of the mast cells I'd had my entire life. All of my crazy reactions—the anaphylaxis from the insect sting, even though I don't have an insect allergy, my many, many episodes of contact dermatitis, the swelling of my arm after the fracture, the post-infectious irritable bowel problems, the urinary urgency that accompanied the rash from the wipe after my hysterectomy, the episodes of chest pain I had every few years—all of these can be caused by mast cell activation syndrome.

Dr. Katz thinks auditory processing disorder exists in part as a result of learning speech sounds through ears infected with otitis media. Well, mast cell activation can cause what's called sterile inflammation—inflammation that exists without a microbial cause. I don't know how many audiologists have even heard of that. I think auditory processing disorder persists because people with APD are hearing over the course of their entire lives through ear canals filled with intermittent sterile inflammation.

In 2014, my body got filled with a laundry list of some of the worst known mast cell triggers. Vancomycin, terbinafine, a ton of anesthesia drugs, SSRIs, and vaccine adjuvants. Huh? Yeah, I didn't say much about vaccines because I'd assumed they were benign. But nothing's benign in a person with an altered immune system. I'd had very few vaccines in my life. I'd had those that were required to enter school in 1980. In 1980, there were only three required vaccines—DTaP, MMR, and polio. I hadn't had any more vaccines until I got the MMR I was told I needed to go to college in 1994. When I looked back at my medical records, I saw I'd gotten the DTaP again in 2010, and I also saw that every time I'd gotten any vaccine, I'd become very sick within days or weeks of it.

I put together a spreadsheet of the ingredients in all the things I've ever reacted to. The ingredient that stood out most is polysorbate 80. My first big exposure to it was in the Lupron. It's an emulsifier in that injection. One study I read showed polysorbate 80 helps transport neurotoxins across the blood-brain barrier. Other studies implicate it in cytotoxicity, or cell death. It's not an inert or benign substance. Huh? Yeah, seriously. And guess what other drugs have polysorbate 80? Depo-Medrol and Zoloft. My abnormal movement symptoms and cognitive problems came back full force after exposure to each of those.

**Why is it that some people can tolerate things like polysorbate 80 and some can't?**

People with more robust microbiomes, people with fully intact blood-brain barriers, people without genetic mutations that disrupt their liver's ability to detoxify the body, they're less likely to be injured. They can tolerate more stuff, or at least it looks like they can in the short term. The long-term effects of most of these ingredients have never been studied.

I'm sure I had a reaction to something in the dilation solution I was given at my eye appointment, but Dr. Bitchy Blob had never heard of that possibility or seen it happen before.

And you know what else? Mast cell activation can cause neuropsychiatric symptoms. Ninety percent of patients with mastocytosis report challenges with things like memory, attention, and focus. There's a doctor—Dr. Theoharis Theoharides—whose research postulates some presentations of autism are actually mast-cell-mediated brain allergies.

**How does that work?**

Neuropeptides can stimulate mast cells. More than half of the histamine in the brain is contained inside mast cells. When mast cells are activated in the brain, they release pro-inflammatory mediators, which include things we've been talking about—histamine, leukotrienes, prostaglandins, and also things like serotonin and cytokines. Cytokines can cause inflammation. Some of these mediators increase the permeability of the blood-brain barrier, so when that happens, you've got a situation where the allergies in the body fuel the allergies in the brain.

Modern autism is a multisystem illness because some of what we're calling autism is *one* presentation of mast cell activation disorder. It's one of many possible outcomes of misbehaving mast cells in the brain. Do you know that PMDD is a common co-occuring condition among autistic women? PMDD and certain types of autism *may be* two facets of the same disease process. Of course you'll find them in the same people! Mast cells also interact with hormones.

Mast cells interact with estrogen. They also interact with something called corticotropin-releasing hormone or CRH. It gets released as part of the stress response. CRH is another trigger for mast cells in the brain. When the mast cells in the brain are triggered, that results in inflammation that manifests as the emotionally overreactive symptoms of autism, so it isn't a huge leap to envision how hormones acting on mast cells in the brain could cause things like mood disorders.

So—big picture—here's what happened: Based on the intersection of the research that currently exists and my history, I've had mast cell problems my whole life. I also had a dearth of healthy microbes from my microbially deficient mother. Sure, I was delivered vaginally, but I came from a woman who was lacking a healthy microbiome, so she couldn't pass on health to me. She only breastfed me for six months, because that's what her doctor told her to do. Even if she'd had healthy microbes to give, six months isn't long enough to get a good dose of them. My pediatrician gave me antibiotics when I had pneumonia as a baby. Then I got the gamma globulin injections. It's possible that I reacted to whatever additives and preservatives were in those injections. Burt told me I wailed for days after each one.

*Why would your mom's microbiome have been so deficient?*

Because she'd never lived in a healthy environment or had a healthy diet. She grew up in a car that her mother drove back and forth between Tucson and Tulsa. They'd briefly stay with my great-grandmother or with one of my grandmother's ever-rotating stable of boyfriends and husbands before returning to the road. My mother's home had been a car—do you get the significance of that? A car saturated with fumes from leaded gas in a time before catalytic converters. My mom was filled with toxins from the time of her birth in 1943. Back then, most people didn't carry the toxic loads many of us carry today. And she was traumatized at an early age. My grandmother and my grandmother's husbands and boyfriends subjected my mom to abuse so unspeakably severe that it makes my childhood look rosy in comparison. Trauma changes your microbes, and not in a good way. She grew up without access to healthy food or any food at all much of the time. She didn't have any of the things a person needs to establish a healthy microbiome. Do you hate her less when you learn that about her? I do.

*Hate her less? I'd say it explains a lot about why she failed as a parent. But I have another question. When you got the fecal transplant to cure the C. diff, wouldn't that have played a role in what happened? Wouldn't the microbiotic transfer from the donor have affected more than just your gut?*

Oh, you're smarter than I thought. Hell yeah, that played a role. It played a huge role. I got my bacteria from Andrew. So, yeah, it cured the C. diff, but it also made me more like him.

*How so?*

You haven't figured that out yet? Andrew's autistic too, old-school congenital Asperger's style. He's introverted as hell. He obsesses over his projects. He obsesses over lots of things—that's why he felt compelled to call me all the time. He's way more anxious than I used to be. Anxiety from social events is literally painful to him. He didn't mean to distract or hurt me by calling all the time. He was just trying to reach out to stop the pain, confusion, and frustration he feels when stressful situations put him into panic mode.

Dealing with people drains him, but he's forced himself to learn and adapt. He's the poster child for how Asperger's presents in males. He's a scientist—how stereotypical can you get? He sees scientific processes in the same way my synesthesia allows me to visualize speech sounds and words. It's a gift of sight and insight that neurotypical people don't have. I got his autism bugs on top of mine, and I got his panic bugs too. Do you know there are studies in mice that show that after fecal transplants, the recipient mouse takes on the personality of the donor mouse. Crazy, huh?

Another key event was the ECT. That gave me a mild brain injury, like a concussion. Research shows that traumatic brain injury contributes to intestinal dysfunction. Brain talks to gut, gut talks to brain. Between the ECT and the antibiotics, I was almost guaranteed to get an infection like C. diff. Concussion also weakens the blood brain barrier.

Are you wondering about my elevated B6 and B12? I went back to Dr. Google for a consult, then I found a brilliant chiropractor who agreed to partner with me in reversing the damage that had happened in 2014. I asked him to help me rule out B12 as a contributing factor in my cognitive problems. By the time I saw him in 2018, my B6 was no longer elevated, and my B12 was at the high end of normal. At my request, he ordered more specific tests to help determine if my B12 was paradoxically low, meaning high in my serum tests because it wasn't getting into my cells where it needed to be. The results of those tests, B12 binding capacity and methylmalonic acid (MMA), showed that while I might have had a problem with B6 and B12 when I saw Dr. Mermer, they were no longer an issue for me. Both were being utilized by my cells.

In September 2018, I saw one more immunologist. He specialized in diagnosing and treating neuropsychiatric conditions that arise from the immune system, including pediatric acute neuropsychiatric disorder associated with streptococcal (PANDAS) and PANS. It was clear to him that something like an autoimmune response had played a role in my regression. Based on my symptoms and the presence of a high level of strep antibodies in tests he ordered, he diagnosed me with adult PANDAS.

The strep antibodies are attacking my brain via a process called molecular mimicry. Strep bacteria hide in the body by covering their cell walls with proteins that look like the proteins of other tissues.

In PANDAS, the antibodies target the basal ganglia because the bacteria cover their cell walls to mimic the appearance of the tissue found in the basal ganglia. The attacks against my basal ganglia explain my oral dyskinesia. PANDAS explains so many things—the obsessive-compulsive disorder that makes me obsess over the shape of silverware, the hyperacusis and other increased sensory sensitivities, the deterioration in my handwriting, and my sudden inability to do basic math.

But PANDAS can also do some of the same things neurological MCAS can do, like cause confusion, rage, anxiety, fear, and panic. PANDAS can also follow a relapsing-remitting pattern, which means it can come and go and fluctuate in severity. I'd noticed that about my symptoms. Sometimes I can think clearly and function well, like when I drove home from Virginia. Sometimes I'm so disoriented I can't even navigate my way around the block. Sometimes I can speak, sometimes I can't. Are these challenges because of PANDAS flares or MCAS flares? Are they both? Where does one end and the other begin? Are the two disease processes intertwined? I have no idea.

Another thing this immunologist did was order more tests of my immune system function—it turns out I am deficient in a subclass of immunity. My body provides me with very little defense against certain infections. And there's something of a paradox in the immune system, where people with immunodeficiencies are at higher risk for developing autoimmune disorders.

I have more answers now, and also more questions. Is PMDD an autoimmune disorder? Does it involve a type of molecular mimicry where antibodies attack progesterone receptors? Have I had low-grade PANDAS my entire life that was exacerbated by hormones, medications or other agents? Do I have the same immunodeficiency now that I had as an infant? Is any of this connected to the connective tissue disorder called Ehlers-Danlos syndrome that runs in my family? I may never learn the answers to these questions.

You know, it's amazing I survived 2014. As an adult, I've lived through many of the mechanisms that account for the increasing autism rates, and I'm here to tell my story. Combine a depleted microbiome with infection and/or environmentally and medically induced hyperstimulation of the immune system, and boom—you get autistic symptoms, allergies, and chronic disease.

This wasn't hard to figure out. All the science is out there for the reading. I get it—the body of medical and scientific literature is enormous. Too big for any human to master. And you doctors are short on time. But I tried to tell you what was happening. I tried to communicate with you, and none of you would listen. You have to release yourselves from the lies, manipulations, and biases that keep your current, harm-inducing practice of medicine alive.

I'm done being told that black is white. I don't care whether the claim comes from my mother, the malignant mental health and medical communities, or the malignant neurodiversity community. Talk to any of them, and you'll hear a lot of lies and bullshit. But none of that matters to me now.

*I'm really glad you've reached this point of liberation and self-acceptance. It's almost like post-traumatic growth.*

Yeah, it is. It's an outcome you all never talk about.

*I have to ask. Since you've broken down, analyzed, and questioned everything, have you questioned your autism diagnosis or autism's existence as a diagnosis?*

Of course I have. It's in *The Unicorn Almanac*, from the syllogism, isn't it? The term "autism" is worthless. It just means the behavioral manifestations of encephalopathy that could derive from any of several causes. It came from the creators of the DSM, who are inextricably immersed in a system that makes zero sense and perpetuates itself out of custom alone.

But I'm done talking about all of this. This whole conversation, the whole course of events I've told you about—it's sucked up years of my life, and the stress of it all has probably taken years *off* my life.

I mean, I appreciate you listening, but this conversation has to come to an end. And you doctors—with your hubris, with your codes of dominance and superiority, with your inability to think critically, with your thin white coat lines—you have to end too.

*What do you mean?*

I mean it's time for you to say goodbye to this world. You didn't notice that the little pill you take for your headaches looked a bit different today, did you?

*What are you . . . are you saying you poisoned me? I don't feel anything.*

Of course you don't feel anything. Do you think that you're real? That you actually exist as a human being? That you can die?

*I—*

No, no don't say "I." There is no "I." No doctor would've ever asked such intelligent, insightful questions. No doctor would've been so patient with me. No doctor would've even pretended to understand me for as long as you have. And I never could have spoken so clearly in response to your questions. I'm not capable of it. I would've gotten more off track and confused. I would've had a meltdown and become nonverbal. This isn't real.

*I did listen. That was real. I'm not judging you. I'm trying to understand. Please. This isn't happening.*

Yes, it is happening. No, it's not happening. Take your pick. How do *you* feel when you realize that what you thought was reality is so unstable? *Are* you real? If you were real, you'd be backtracking. You'd be thinking, *Oh shit, she is borderline. She is nuts.* But I'm not. I understand consequences. I understand them better than most people. I think things through. I'm not impulsive—well, not for the most part. The thing is, you're not real. You're a figment of my imagination. You're a literary device. I can't kill you. You're an idea—a really fucking bad idea.

*No, I'm—*

I'm going to let you dissolve now. You're going to dissolve into little particles. Each particle is going to carry away bits of my anger and bits of my pain—anger and pain over how there's rarely justice in one lifetime. Anger over how the statute ran out, and I'll never be compensated for what you all did to me. Anger over how you all played into one another's lies until you destroyed my body and brain in 2014. Each particle is going to take away a little bit of that pain.

*No! No, it won't. Killing me won't stop the pain.*

Still working through that denial, doc? Ha-ha. You weren't listening. I can't kill you. I've handed you over to these other people, to these readers. You'll be alive for as long as they're thinking of you. And you'll stand accountable to their judgment. That's how there'll be justice. The statute can't stop that.

*Don't! This is cra—*

Relax. It's just your brain swelling. Just a little grey and white matter pressing against your skull. It's all in your head. Relax into it. You're dissolving into the light of truth. The light of compassion. You're human, just like me.

You yield to authority, systemic and individual. You relied on ideas that were supposed to be trustworthy, and in doing so you stopped trusting your own judgment. You refused to believe the truth of what you saw happening in front of you. You thought your education and reputation would protect you. Ha! Nothing will protect you. You're flawed. I'm flawed. We're all flawed. And you're forgiven. And I'm free.